Fast Facts for HEALTH PROMOTION IN NURSING: *Promoting Wellness in a Nutshell* (Miller)

Fast Facts for STROKE CARE NURSING: *An Expert Guide in a Nutshell* (Morrison)

Fast Facts for the MEDICAL OFFICE NURSE: *What You Really Need to Know in a Nutshell* (Richmeier)

Fast Facts for the PEDIATRIC NURSE: *An Orientation Guide in a Nutshell* (Rupert, Young)

Fast Facts About the GYNECOLOGICAL EXAM FOR NURSE PRACTITIONERS: *Conducting the GYN Exam in a Nutshell* (Secor, Fantasia)

Fast Facts for the STUDENT NURSE: *Nursing Student Success in a Nutshell* (Stabler-Haas)

Fast Facts for CAREER SUCCESS IN NURSING: *Making the Most of Mentoring in a Nutshell* (Vance)

Fast Facts for the TRIAGE NURSE: *An Orientation and Care Guide in a Nutshell* (Visser, Montejano, Grossman)

Fast Facts for DEVELOPING A NURSING ACADEMIC PORTFOLIO: *What You Really Need to Know in a Nutshell* (Wittmann-Price)

Fast Facts for the CLASSROOM NURSING INSTRUCTOR: *Classroom Teaching in a Nutshell* (Yoder-Wise, Kowalski)

Forthcoming FAST FACTS Books

Fast Facts for TESTING AND EVALUATION IN NURSING: *Teaching Skills in a Nutshell* (Dusaj)

Fast Facts for the CLINICAL NURSE MANAGER: *Managing a Changing Workplace in a Nutshell, 2e* (Fry)

Fast Facts for the CARDIAC SURGERY NURSE: *Caring for Cardiac Surgery Patients in a Nutshell, 2e* (Hodge)

Fast Facts About the NURSING PROFESSION: *Historical Perspectives in a Nutshell* (Hunt)

Fast Facts for the HOSPICE NURSE: *A Concise Guide to End-of-Life Care* (Wright)

Visit www.springerpub.com to order.

FAST FACTS FOR THE SCHOOL NURSE

School Nursing in a Nutshell

Janice Loschiavo, MSN, RN, HNCSN, is an adjunct instructor at William Paterson University Graduate Nursing Division and at Caldwell College in the Education/Nursing Division. She had 26 years of experience as a school nurse before retiring from those positions in 2007. Ms. Loschiavo has received recognition for excellence both in teaching and as a school nurse, including the New Jersey Distinguished Alumni Award (2014), the Governor's Teacher Recognition Award in 2006–2007, the nominee for Disney Teacher of the Year (2002), the New Jersey State School Nurse of the Year (1994–1995), the Bergen County School Nurse of the Year (1994–1995), and the state nominee for National School Nurse of the Year (1994–1995). While a school nurse, she was responsible for participating in Child Study Team meetings, maintaining health records, conducting health screenings, and providing first aid to students; teaching health classes; conducting faculty inservice training (anaphylaxis, child abuse, and first aid); organizing health fairs; running workshops for teachers and parents; and serving as liaison to the Division of Youth and Family Services. Ms. Loschiavo contributed to the recently published book *Health Counseling: A Microskills Approach for Counselors, Educators, and School Nurses*, Second Edition, edited by Richard Blonna. *Advance for Nurses* published her article, "Considering School Nursing?" in January 2013.

FAST FACTS FOR THE SCHOOL NURSE

School Nursing in a Nutshell

Second Edition

Janice Loschiavo, MSN, RN, HNCSN

SPRINGER PUBLISHING COMPANY

NEW YORK

Springer Publishing Company, LLC
11 West 42nd Street
New York, NY 10036
www.springerpub.com

Acquisitions Editor: Margaret Zuccarini
Production Editor: Kris Parrish
Composition: S4Carlisle Publishing Services

ISBN: 978-0-8261-2876-8
e-book ISBN: 978-0-8261-2877-5

16 17 18 / 5 4

The author and the publisher of this Work have made every effort to use sources believed to be reliable to provide information that is accurate and compatible with the standards generally accepted at the time of publication. The author and publisher shall not be liable for any special, consequential, or exemplary damages resulting, in whole or in part, from the readers' use of, or reliance on, the information contained in this book. The publisher has no responsibility for the persistence or accuracy of URLs for external or third-party Internet websites referred to in this publication and does not guarantee that any content on such websites is, or will remain, accurate or appropriate.

Library of Congress Cataloging-in-Publication Data

Loschiavo, Janice, author.
  Fast facts for the school nurse : school nursing in a nutshell / Janice Loschiavo.—Second edition.
    p. ; cm.
  Includes bibliographical references and index.
  ISBN 978-0-8261-2876-8—ISBN 0-8261-2876-9—ISBN 978-0-8261-2877-5 (e-book)
  I. Title.
  [DNLM: 1. School Nursing—methods. 2. Nurse's Practice Patterns. WY 113]
  RJ247
  371.7'12—dc23
                                                                    2014043678

Printed in the United States of America by Gasch Printing.

*This book is dedicated to all
school nurses—past, present, and future.
May we always remember—
Children cannot interrupt your work.
They are your work.*

Contents

Part I: Health Problems and Nursing Management: Making the Change

Part II: Health Appraisal: Health Promotion and Disease Prevention

Part III: Professional Issues

Foreword

School nursing is noble work and a recognized specialty within the profession of nursing. Its origin can be traced to the dawn of the 19th century, with Lillian Wald and her founding of the Henry Street Settlement in New York City. Wald and her nurses were politically astute and tenacious in advocating for the health of the community. Their legacy was the establishment of school nursing as a vital part of the community.

School nurses strive to deliver to educators students who are in optimum condition for learning. The mission of the educational system is doomed to failure without the knowledge and skills of school nurses who intervene to solve actual health problems, manage chronic diseases, and promote health and healthful lifestyles. All of this is accomplished within the orientation of the community and the primary system for care for most children—the family.

Of course, success is impossible unless the behaviors of healthful living are instilled in the students themselves. The ultimate goal of school nursing is self-care and personal understanding of the meaning of health and wellness. It starts with having students appreciate the health legacy of the family and how investing in a healthful lifestyle will serve them well throughout life—and further, how once lost, health may be difficult to recapture. School nurses convey such understanding through role modeling and the education process. First and foremost, a school nurse is a teacher.

The work of a school nurse is not for the faint of heart, especially in today's milieu of social diversity, complex medical treatments, and the expectation that, whenever possible, children with special needs will be mainstreamed to promote lives as close to being normal as possible. For most school nurses, every day is a cacophony of special needs, each to be resolved, each unique and different from every other in its cause and solution. Modern times have brought more attention to student needs: autism spectrum disorders, childhood obesity, drug use (both prescribed and illegal), problems of sexuality and mental health, school violence, child abuse, and cultural diversity, to name a few. It is clear that these issues have to be approached within a team context, but each is inextricably associated with health and demands the holistic perspective that characterizes nursing.

Beyond the human problems that dominate the work of school nursing, there are the legal, ethical, and institutional policies that represent both assistance and obstacles to bringing the best of nursing science to students. *Fast Facts for the School Nurse* is a virtual compendium of situations that school nurses encounter in their practice. It will direct school nurses to the answers for many questions and to wiser counsel when a dilemma seems unsolvable. It is a reference for school nurses authored by a school nurse of publicly acclaimed distinction who brings a lifetime of experience to these pages.

Lucille A. Joel, EdD, RN, FAAN
Professor, College of Nursing
Rutgers, The State University of New Jersey
Newark, New Jersey

Preface

If you are a school nurse, you likely have been asked the same con-
descending question from nursing colleagues that I have: "How
could you have gone from being a fabulous emergency department
or intensive care nurse to being a *school nurse*? All you do now is
put on Band-Aids and give out tooth-fairy necklaces."

If you do not have a good answer, I will give you mine: "As a
school nurse and health teacher, my challenge will be to *prevent* a
disease, accident, or illness from occurring in the first place. If I do
my job well, there will be far fewer patients in emergency departments and intensive care units."

BACKGROUND

Today's schools are very different from those of the past. They
must be, because today's students are also quite different. Children today face challenges unique to the times. They may come
from the growing number of unstable homes. Highly addictive, illegal drugs are now easily available. Sexually transmitted diseases
have always been a concern, but AIDS can carry a death sentence.
Other risk factors such as obesity and sedentary lifestyles are not
only unhealthful but can also lead to childhood unhappiness.
Cultural diversity and environmental issues contribute to feelings
of fear and isolation. Mainstreamed children with special needs
are particularly vulnerable and in need of much support. All of
these factors and many more can interfere with a student's ability
to learn.

The schools and the people within them often provide the only stability in some children's lives. Therefore, it makes sense that school personnel be educated to recognize the turmoil in such children's lives and offer needed guidance.

It is no secret that an ill, unhappy child simply cannot learn. This book will help school nurses recognize a wide range of health issues and the ever-expanding role that they have in prevention and treatment. In doing so, the school nurse will free children to learn and grow in a safe, nurturing academic environment.

THE PURPOSE OF THIS BOOK

The reader will find this book useful for two purposes. First, it is a quick-reference guide for both the novice and the experienced school nurse who wishes to keep abreast of new information. The special health issues section will be particularly helpful in preventing and dealing with some of today's most prevalent health issues.

This book can also serve as a supplemental textbook for nurses who are enrolled in college or university programs of study for state certification or who are preparing to take the examination for national certification through the National Board for the Certification of School Nurses. This book includes relevant information about the five components included in the exam and in the courses that must be taken: health problems and nursing management, health appraisal, health promotion and disease prevention, professional issues, and special health issues.

ORGANIZATION OF THIS BOOK

Part I covers basic elements of the specialty of school nursing. Part II addresses school nurses' role in student assessment and health counseling. Part III discusses professional responsibilities of school nurses. Part IV examines some of the most important health issues that affect students today and what school nurses in their role of nurse and health teacher can do to prevent, recognize early, and manage these issues in the school setting.

NEW FEATURES OF THIS SECOND EDITION

I am most excited about two new features included in this second edition. You will note continued references to the *Healthy People 2020* initiatives. *Healthy People* has been expanded to encompass numerous areas relevant to our practice. School nurses need to work in concert with the rest of the nation to help meet target objectives by raising the level of wellness one child at a time. Where relevant, I have added the *Healthy People 2020* objectives for you to reference. I have also added a chapter that deals specifically with a range of current issues that frustrate and challenge us as school nurses. I hope that my personal insights and suggestions will ease your concerns and free you to spend more time directly working with children.

THE AUTHOR'S GOALS

My goals in writing this book are simple. I wish to share my passion for school nursing and to help my colleagues recognize that their school nursing careers are unique opportunities for helping students and the larger community.

I wish you well and hope that you will find this book not only an essential guide, but also a comfort as you meet the exciting professional challenges of school nursing.

Janice Loschiavo

Acknowledgments

I thank Margaret Zuccarini, Publisher of Nursing at Springer Publishing Company, for recognizing the need for a book such as this. Margaret also "held my hand" through the writing process and patiently answered my many questions.

I thank my friend Lucille Joel for her encouragement throughout my school nurse career and for serving as such a wonderful role model—not only as a nurse but as a wife, mother, and grandmother, as well.

I thank my son Rick, and son-in-law John Ferro, for their technical insight in helping me put the manuscript together.

I also thank my many school nurse colleagues, especially Mary Ellen Bolton and Jan Halder, who continue to impress me with their knowledge and, in doing so, have kept me humble.

I thank my three children—Lori, Jill, and Rick—for demonstrating kindness and maturity beyond their years when they so often had to share their mother. I thank them also for the gift of grandchildren: Ryan, Ashley, Richard, Luke, Preston, and Austin. These bright, beautiful babies keep me focused on what truly matters in life.

Most of all, I thank my husband Rich. Over these past months Rich has learned to tolerate piles of papers and a very distracted, preoccupied wife. After 47 years of marriage, he continues to "hold my hand" and heart as well.

I

Health Problems and Nursing Management

Making the Change

Bed Baths to Band-Aids

What the School Nurse *Really* Does

You might have a number of reasons for wanting a career as a school nurse. Maybe you feel that you are no longer physically or emotionally up to the demands of hospital work. Perhaps you want shorter workdays and work years so that you can spend more time at home, or you are simply tired of being away from your family on weekends and holidays. These certainly are valid reasons for wanting a change.

There may be other, more subtle reasons why you are considering a career as a school nurse. You may be frustrated by caring for patients who are ill because of poor lifestyle choices, interested in helping prevent diseases and accidents, ready to work independently, or seeking a greater professional challenge. If these issues resonate with you, I invite you to join me in the role of school nurse/teacher of health. Together with our colleagues, we can elevate the quality of health care for each child. In doing so, we also can raise the level of wellness for schools, communities, and the nation itself.

In this chapter, you will learn:

1. The definition of school nursing
2. The history of school nursing and how it is rooted in public health
3. The components of a *coordinated school health program*

4. The unique roles and goals of school nurses
5. The importance of the *Healthy People* initiatives
6. The three levels of prevention.

DEFINITION

The National Association of School Nurses (NASN) defines *school nursing* as:

> A specialized practice of professional nursing that advances the well-being, academic success, and life-long achievement and health of students. To that end, school nurses facilitate positive student responses to normal development; promote health and safety including a healthy environment; intervene with actual and potential health problems; provide case management services; and actively collaborate with others to build student and family capacity for adaptation, self-management, self advocacy, and learning. (NASN, 2010)

Simply put, school nurses support student achievement through wellness. We are nurses *and* teachers who work to prevent and control illnesses so that students can learn to their greatest potential.

HISTORY

Early Beginnings

Before the 19th century, the United States had little in the way of a formal health care delivery system. Births, injuries, illnesses, and deaths were dealt with at home, and caring for family members was an accepted part of everyday life. In the late 1800s, thousands of people immigrated to New York from rural areas of the United States and from Europe. These people were often poor, homeless, hungry, very sick, and far from relatives and friends. With only a fragment of a health care delivery system in place, there was no one to tend to their many needs. It was also around this time that New York City enacted legislation requiring students to attend school. The prevalence of contagious diseases, already high in the community, increased as students gathered in school settings. The most common contagious diseases of the time—tuberculosis, pediculosis, ringworm, impetigo, and conjunctivitis—were all transmitted in crowded and unsanitary conditions.

Although compulsory school attendance was a huge step forward in education, it was a recipe for disaster because of the health concerns. It was not unusual for a child to be repeatedly exposed, infected, and excluded from school for the same disease. A child could be permanently truant because of a small, curable lesion. Poor children often left school by the age of 14 to take their place in the workforce or to watch their younger siblings while their parents earned a living.

The health needs of the populace were so overwhelming that they presented a tremendous threat to the growth of the city. One woman chose to do something about it. Lillian Wald was a bright young lady from an affluent family who had graduated from the New York Hospital School of Nursing. One day, while she was teaching a class to immigrant women, a young girl asked her to help her very ill mother. Wald made a house call and was appalled by the living conditions of the poor people whom she encountered. She found large families living in single rooms shared with boarders. All the tenants in the building used one toilet, which had no door and seldom worked. Wald was ashamed to be part of a society that allowed conditions like this to exist, and she committed herself to improving the lives of these poor people.

Wald, along with friend and colleague Mary Brewster, founded the Visiting Nurse Service of New York in 1893 with funding from philanthropists and friends. By January of 1894, the two had visited more than 125 families. One year later, Wald moved herself and seven other nurses to 265 Henry Street, a tenement in one of the poorest neighborhoods of New York City. There, she founded the renowned Henry Street Settlement, which still exists today.

The Henry Street Settlement

The Henry Street Settlement was the top floor of the house where the nurses lived and worked. From their home, they were able to easily access those in greatest need and their patients could reach them. Their patients were referred to as "neighbors."

Wald wanted the Settlement to be a place where all were welcome. She felt strongly that people had to be viewed in totality. Meals were served, the homeless were sheltered, and piano lessons were given to the poor in the dining room. Wald recognized that even the indigent had needs for creative expression. Under her direction, the seeds of many social changes were planted. Wald advocated for child labor laws, park and playground construction, special education, women's suffrage, housing codes, and the profession of school nursing. She was a founding member of the National Association for the Advancement of Colored People and supported funding for "fresh air" programs that would become the Fresh Air Fund.

The Experiment

In 1896, the New York City Department of Health set about addressing the high percentage of absent children in public schools. One hundred and fifty of the finest physicians were hired to spend 1 hour a day inspecting schoolchildren. Their focus was to exclude sick children from school. There was no follow-up or teaching of positive health habits. Once children were excluded, they simply did not return to school—ever. Meanwhile, in just a few years, the Henry Street Settlement had grown. Wald was not only a visionary nurse, but also a savvy politician. Once she became aware of the failure of the physicians' work, she made an offer to New York City's schools chancellor. Wald proposed to provide a nurse who would work in four of the schools with the greatest number of absent and medically excluded children. If the absentee rate significantly decreased, the city would then pay to have a school nurse in every school.

On October 1, 1902, Lina Rogers, one of the eight nurses from the Henry Street Settlement, started her job. She spent 1 hour a day at each school, with a total enrollment of 8,671 students. With limited space and almost no supplies, she dressed wounds, treated conjunctivitis, cleaned skin infections, and excluded children from school when necessary. However, this time, the excluded children received follow-up visits in their homes, where parents were educated about health issues. Rogers recognized the needs of both patient and family; she made referrals, and follow-up care was provided. Children recovered, returned to school, and were able to learn. The program was so successful that 25 more nurses were soon hired. Within 1 year, absenteeism decreased by 90% and New York City became the first municipality in the world to take financial responsibility for children's health while they were in school. One young, humble nurse working in deplorable conditions had succeeded where 150 prominent physicians had failed. Why? She recognized the complexity of the health needs of individuals and offered herself as a nurse, teacher, and friend.

School nursing has its roots in public health. Nursing pioneers recognized that caring for children in the school setting was an excellent means of controlling disease and that children needed to be well enough to attend school so education could take place. Working conditions were initially deplorable but improved once the school nurses' work became recognized and respected.

Clinical Snapshot

Catherine was thrilled to be hired as a school nurse immediately after graduation. She was not so thrilled when she saw her tiny, hot, inaccessible office with no bathroom nearby. After the initial shock, Catherine rolled up her sleeves and began to work within the system to improve the health office atmosphere and establish herself as an important presence.

As you plan your school nurse practice, remember our public health roots and accept that although you may have less than perfect working conditions, you can still be an effective school nurse and a dynamic health teacher.

Years of Growth

In the years that followed the New York City experiment, the role of school nurses expanded in concert with the needs of the students and the community. Children were still evaluated and excluded from school when warranted, but the responsibility for health began to shift to the home. School nurses enabled this transition through education. Health education began to emerge as a separate discipline, and certified school nurses were the major force in making the necessary changes.

As World War II loomed, the focus was on national security. Healthy men were needed to serve quickly. Unfortunately, one fourth of all draftees were rejected because of the residual effects of preventable childhood illnesses or malnutrition. It became clear that there were lingering aftereffects of childhood illnesses that, in many instances, could have been avoided with preventive education, early detection, and prompt treatment.

Recognizing these health issues, school nurses began to develop programs and work with teachers to incorporate them

TABLE 1.1 School Nursing Historical Timeline

1892	London Amy Hughes is hired to investigate the nutritional status of schoolchildren in the school setting. This is the first recorded employment of a school nurse.
1893	Belgium Brussels is the first city to employ a school physician and establish organized, citywide inspection of schools.
1894	Boston School health services are initiated to identify and exclude students with serious communicable diseases such as pertussis, measles, mumps, scarlet fever, and parasitic diseases, including lice, ringworm, and scabies.
1902	New York The Henry Street Settlement is organized, modeled after an English program. Lillian Wald, head nurse, appoints Lina Rogers as the nation's first school nurse. The goal is to decrease absenteeism following implementation of mandatory school attendance. Between 1902 and 1903 the number of absentees decreases from 10,567 to 1,101. Twenty-five more nurses are then hired and paid by the New York City Board of Education.
1920s	This decade sees the expansion of the school nurse's role. Health education is added and medical examinations begin in schools to identify physical defects.
1930s	Individual states begin to require specific education for school nurse practice.
1940s	War is present in much of the world. Leaders in the United States realize the importance of the maximum degree of health for all to serve in the armed forces and support the country at home. Health as a school subject begins to include an emphasis on physical fitness. Educators recognize the correlation between health teaching and practice.
1950s	The role of the school nurse is expanded to focus on prevention. Screenings in dental health, vision, and hearing are followed up and fewer students are left with chronic diseases. Health counseling is introduced.

(continued)

TABLE 1.1 School Nursing Historical Timeline (*continued*)

1960	Some states require nurses to have teaching degrees.
1965	Federal laws begin to take shape ensuring that all children, handicapped or not, are appropriately educated. These laws further strengthen the position of the school nurse, whose presence now is required to perform treatments and give medications in the school setting. These laws continue to be revised, renamed, and enhanced to further benefit all children with special needs.
1968	The National Education Association (NEA) establishes the Department of School Nurses (DSN). A nationwide survey is conducted to establish school nurse credentials for each state. The DSN begins to form committees, develop policies, and elect officers.
1979	The DSN separates from NEA to form the National Association of School Nurses (NASN), which now serves as the hub for all the state organizations.
Today	School nursing continues to flourish as a separate discipline. Through NASN, school nurses partner with national health organizations, publish a journal and reference books, formulate position statements, and hold nationwide conventions to disseminate information and foster communication. NASN also employs a Washington, DC–based representative to lobby for school nursing issues and interact with Congress on the organization's behalf.

into the curriculum. Classes in nutrition were taught to students and parents. Screenings were done and children with vision or hearing problems were referred and treated. School health services expanded into a comprehensive program, with the school nurse assuming more of a teaching role.

COMPONENTS OF A COORDINATED SCHOOL HEALTH PROGRAM

The eight-component model of a school health program was originally proposed by Allensworth and Kolbe (1987). Their expanded perspective encouraged links within the school community and suggested that time and resources could be better utilized if school health programs were coordinated and comprehensive. A coordinated school health program is intended to serve as an interactive framework across school settings. The eight components are:

1. Health education
2. Physical education
3. Health services
4. Nutrition services
5. Mental health and social services
6. Healthful and safe school environment
7. Health promotion for staff
8. Parent/family and community involvement

ROLES AND GOALS OF THE SCHOOL NURSE

Wold (1981) summarized the position of school nurse as having five roles and goals:

1. *Manager of health care within the school health program:* To participate in planning, implementation, and evaluation of the school health program.
2. *Deliverer of health services:* To deliver needed health services to the client system using systematic processes to assess needs, plan interventions, and evaluate outcomes so that high-level wellness can be achieved.
3. *Advocate for health rights of children:* To act as an advocate for health rights of children and their families within the school setting and between the school and community.
4. *Counselor for health concerns of children, families, and staff:* To provide health counseling and guidance for the client system on an individual basis or within a group setting.
5. *Educator for school/community health concerns:* To participate in health education program activities for children, youth, school personnel, and the community.

In a revised position statement (2011a) the NASN and the American Academy of Pediatrics (AAP) together updated and further elaborated on the role of the school nurse:

- *School nurses facilitate normal development and positive student response to interventions.* The school nurse develops plans for student care based on the nursing process.

- *School nurses provide leadership in promoting health and safety, including a healthy environment.* The school nurse is a leader in the development of school safety plans to address bullying, school violence, and the full range of emergencies that may occur at school.
- *School nurses provide quality health care and intervene with actual and potential health problems.* Students often have multiple needs that should be examined in order for the student to be successful.
- *School nurses use clinical judgment in providing case management services.*
- *School nurses develop Individualized Healthcare plans (IHPs) in nursing language to direct nursing care for students as well as Emergency Care Plans (ECPs) written in lay language to guide the response of unlicensed personnel in a health-related emergency.*
- *School nurses actively collaborate with others to build student and family capacity for adaptation, self-management, self-advocacy, and learning.* The school nurse is essential to the educational teams, such as Section 504 or Child Study (Individualized Education Plan), so that health barriers to learning can be reduced (U.S. Department of Health and Human Services, 2010).

HEALTHY PEOPLE INITIATIVES

It has long been recognized that the health of each individual is linked to the health of the community and the health of the community is the foundation for the health of the nation.

In 1979, *Healthy People* was initiated by the U.S. Department of Health and Human Services. It is a comprehensive, nationwide health promotion and disease prevention agenda. It represents a set of national 10-year goals and objectives developed to improve the health of all Americans. These objectives were written after referencing over 8,000 comments from diverse individuals and organizations. *Healthy People* now guides the country by providing a list of priorities for each ensuing decade. At the completion of each decade, the objectives are evaluated and new ones developed to meet the needs of the changing world. In 1990, 226 health objectives were listed. Today, the *Healthy People 2020* initiative encompasses over 1,200 areas to improve our nation's health.

Healthy People is grounded in the principle that setting objectives and monitoring progress can motivate action and behavior change. *Healthy People 2010* saw 23% of its objectives met or exceeded and 48% moved toward the target goal. Thus far, it is estimated that the country has made progress toward or met 71% of its *Healthy People* targets. (Centers for Disease Control and Prevention, 2010). *Please see Appendix A for all* Healthy People 2020 *topics.*

Today's school nurse must be cognizant of ever-changing world needs and respectful of the data presented. With this information we can develop timely health programs for our schools and influence policy making in the communities we live and work within.

Healthy People 2020 Objective

Educational and Community-Based Programs, 5.1

Increase the proportion of elementary, middle, and high schools that have a full-time, registered, school nurse-to-student ratio of at least 1:750 from 40.6% in 2006 to 44.7%.

LEVELS OF PREVENTION

School nurses differ from hospital nurses in that we deal with prevention, as opposed to intervention. We seek to prevent health problems through education. In the hospital we intervene because a problem already exists and must be fixed. There are three levels of prevention to be considered in the delivery of health care in school settings: primary, secondary, and tertiary (Wold, 1981).

Primary Prevention

Primary prevention takes place before an illness or injury occurs. Its measures include health education, basic hygiene, immunizations, and healthful lifestyle practices. This level of prevention is the most cost effective and efficient.

Secondary Prevention

Once a person is affected by disease, an accident has occurred, or a health issue becomes apparent, school nurses seek to render a diagnosis and offer prompt, effective treatment. By doing so, we stop the progression and lessen the effects of the problem. Measures include first aid, vision or hearing referrals, and exclusion from school.

Tertiary Prevention

Tertiary prevention is needed for students with existing disabilities for which rehabilitation is expected. The goal is to allow students the maximum school experience in the least restrictive environment while dealing with their disabilities.

Prevention Versus Intervention

Primary and secondary prevention are the keys to cost-effective, comprehensive health care. Prevention through education is the focus of the school nurse and the main way in which we differ from our nursing colleagues. Tertiary prevention is costly in terms of time, money, and pain.

FAST FACTS in a NUTSHELL

All school nurses must adapt to the individual needs of their students and community. Allow yourself the opportunity to explore different types of school settings. You may be surprised to learn that you have strengths you previously did not recognize.

Clinical Snapshot

School nurse Catherine was dismayed when she was assigned to the high school instead of the elementary school where a nurse had retired. Recognizing that the school district and superintendent had this option, she resigned herself to accepting the high school position. Several years later when Catherine was offered the elementary position, she decided to stay at the high school. Catherine found she enjoyed working with older students and honestly felt that this is where she was needed most.

2

Educational Preparation for the School Nurse

Now that you have decided to take on this new professional challenge, you will need to prepare yourself—mentally, physically, and academically. This preparation is important and will not be easy. If it were, many more would choose school nursing.

Begin by exploring your state regulations for school nurse practice. Once you know what must be done, spend some time in a school health office before you invest your money and commit to a career that might be quite different from what you previously perceived.

In this chapter, you will learn:

1. The National Association of School Nurses' recommended minimum educational criteria
2. The requirements for educational preparation as a school nurse in your state
3. The requirements for national school nurse certification
4. The scope of practice of the school nurse
5. School nursing subspecialties
6. The future of school nursing

NATIONAL ASSOCIATION OF SCHOOL NURSES' EDUCATIONAL RECOMMENDATIONS

School nurses are part of two disciplines: nursing and education. The National Association of School Nurses (NASN) in a 2012 position statement established minimum educational criteria for the school nurse:

> It is the position of NASN that every school-aged child deserves a school nurse who is a graduate of a baccalaureate degree program from an accredited college or university and licensed by that state as a registered nurse. These requirements are the minimal preparation for the skills needed at the entry level of school nursing practice. In addition, NASN supports state certification, where required, and promotes national certification of school nurses through the National Board for Certification of School Nurses.

FAST FACTS in a NUTSHELL

In 1791, the Tenth Amendment to the Constitution was passed, giving the rights of education to the individual states, *not* the federal government. This means that states that are geographically close may have entirely different educational requirements.

Clinical Snapshot

Mary Beth was relieved to learn that she only needed a few credits in addition to her bachelor's degree to become certified as a school nurse in her state. She had never worked in a school but liked the schedule, which would allow her to be home with her children in the afternoons and in summer.

Before jumping into this new challenge, Mary Beth should be certain that she fully understands what a school nurse does. The role of a school nurse might actually be quite different from her perception, and it may not be work she enjoys. It would be prudent if she offered to substitute for a while to be certain this is what she wants to do before enrolling in certification courses and spending valuable time and money.

Mary Beth must also look objectively at the change in salary. The work day and year may be shorter but the pay will probably be less, as well.

Educational Preparation

With few exceptions, school nurses work independently. Their abilities, education, experience, and job performance must be exceptional. It is essential that school nurses know the specific regulations in their state so they practice within the law.

═══════════════════════════════════FAST FACTS in a NUTSHELL

As the school nurse's role continues to expand, initiatives and laws are developed that support and guide our practice. These laws are continually changing to meet the needs of our ever-changing society.

Clinical Snapshot

School nurse Kathy worked for years at a school in her home district. When her husband was transferred out of state, Kathy sought employment in the new school system. She was dismayed to learn that she had to return to school for further coursework to qualify for employment.

All states require some specific preparation to work in a school. Many go beyond this to require a bachelor's degree and certification. Certification is a commitment of value, and the burden is on states to define and demand a minimum but appropriate level of preparation for their school health practitioners (Schwab & Gelfman, 2001, p. 499).

An extensive study of the individual state regulations for school nurse practice was conducted by Praeger and Zimmerman (2009). The following is a summary of their findings:

- All states authorize registered nurses to provide health services; 30 states require state school nurse credentials.
- Thirty-one states have health department staff provide school nurse coverage.
- Twenty-three states mention licensed or vocational practical nurses as being able to provide school services, but their practice might be limited.
- A baccalaureate degree for the registered nurse is specified in 25 states, with 9 of those stipulating that it must be in nursing.
- Twenty-seven states require a school nurse credential, whether it be a license or certificate, to be recognized as a school nurse.

- Twenty-nine states have the department of education authorize the title of school nurse and 23 receive authorization from the local school districts. Table 2.1 contains an outline of all data contained in this study.

National School Nurse Certification

National school nurse certification is offered through the National Board for Certification of School Nurses (NBCSN). To be eligible to sit for the NBCSN examination, the candidate must meet these requirements:

- Possess a valid license as a registered nurse in the United States
- Have completed a baccalaureate degree in nursing or a health-related field
- Have 3 years of experience as a school nurse (NBCSN, 2012)

The better prepared the school nurse is, the better she will function in the school setting. Even when a degree or specific courses are not required by the state, it is important for the school nurse to continuously seek educational opportunities to enhance her job performance.

FAST FACTS in a NUTSHELL

We have all worked with wonderful nurses, but we also know of some nurses who are not so wonderful. A work situation is often manageable because we focus on each other's greater strengths and work as a team. In a school setting, there is no other nurse or team member; thus, it is not enough to be a satisfactory school nurse. Every school nurse must be an outstanding school nurse.

Clinical Snapshot

Debbie is finding that the most difficult part of her new school nurse job is the lack of nurse colleagues. The nature of the position separates her from the other teachers and staff. Debbie will need to find school nurse role models within the district or county and establish relationships with these nurses. Although they cannot work alongside her, these are the colleagues who will mentor and support her.

TABLE 2.1 State Regulations for School Nurse Practice

State	Authorized to Provide Health Services in Schools	Criteria for Becoming SN	Source of Title	SN Protected Title	SN Mandate	Renewal Requirement
AL	LPN, RN, MD, U	LPN, RN	Dist		X	
AK	RN*, PHN, MD	RN*, Bacc-Ed	DoE	X		Ed
AZ	RN*	RN*	BoN	X		BSN/Ed/CE
AR	LPN, RN, HD, MD, U	RN*	Dist		X	Ed
CA	RN*, MD, D	RN*-Bacc-Ed	DoE	X		Ed, exp
CO	LPN, RN, RN*, HD, MD, D, U	RN*-Bacc-exp-NC	DoE	X		Ed/CE
CT	LPN, RN, RN*, MD, D	RN-exp-Ed/CE	Dist	X	X	CE
DC	LPN, RN, HD, MD, U	LPN, RN	DoH		X	
DE	RN*	RN*-BSN/BaccSchNsg.exp	DoE	X	X	CE/Ed
FL	LPN, RN, HD, MD, D, U	LPN, RN	Dist			
GA	LPN, RN, HD	LPN, RN	Dist		X	
HI	PHN, U	PHN	DoH			
ID	RN*	RN*	DoE	X		Bacc/ED-exp-tech

(continued)

TABLE 2.1 State Regulations for School Nurse Practice (continued)

State	Authorized to Provide Health Services in Schools	Criteria for Becoming SN	Source of Title	SN Protected Title	SN Mandate	Renewal Requirement
IL	RN*, MD	RN*-Bacc-Ed-exp	DoE	X	X	CE
IN	LPN, RN*	RN*-BSN	DoE	X	X	Ed
IA	RN, RN*	RN, RN*-Bacc, RN*-BSN-exp	Dist, DoE	X	X	Ed
KS	LPN, RN*	RN*-BSN	DoE	X	X	Ed
KY	LPN, RN, RN*, MD	RN*-exp, RN*-Bacc-exp/NC	DoE	X		Ed/CE, exp
LA	RN*, U	RN*-exp, RN*-Bacc-exp	DoE	X	X	Ed, exp
ME	RN*, MD	RN*-Bacc-exp	DoE	X	X	Ed/CE
MD	RN, HD, MD, U	RN-Ed	Dist, DoH			CE
MA	RN*, MD	RN*-BSN-Ed/NC	DoE	X	X	Ed, NC
MI	RN*, HD, U	RN*-exp-Ed/Bacc	DoE	X		Ed
MN	RN*, PHN	RN*-BSN-PHN	DoE	X	X	CE
MS	LPN, RN, HD, MD	RN	Dist		X	
MO	LPN, RN, HD, MD	RN	Dist		X	
MT	LPN, RN, HD, MD, D, U	LPN, RN	Dist			

(continued)

TABLE 2.1 State Regulations for School Nurse Practice (continued)						
State	Authorized to Provide Health Services in Schools	Criteria for Becoming SN	Source of Title	SN Protected Title	SN Mandate	Renewal Requirement
NE	LPN, RN, RN*, HD, MD, D, U	RN*-Ed	DoE	X		Ed
NY	RN*, HD, U	RN*Bacc-Ed/NC, RN*-BSN	DoE	X		
NH	LPN, RN, HD, MD, D, U	RN	Dist	X	X	
NJ	RN, RN*, MD, U	RN, RN*-Bacc-Ed	Dist, DoE	X	X	Ed/CE
NM	LPN*, RN*, HD, MD	LPN*-exp, RN*	DoE	X		Competency
NY	RN, RN*, HD, MD, D, U	RN, RN-Ed, RN*-Bacc-Ed	Dist, DoH, DoE	X		Ed/CE
NC	RN	RN	Dist	X	X	NC
ND	LPN, RN, HD, MD, D, U	LPN, RN	Dist		X	
OH	RN*, HD, MD, D, U	RN*-Bacc-ed	DoE	X	X	
OK	LPN, RN, RN*, HD, U	RN*	DoE	X	X	
OR	RN, RN*, HD, MD, D	RN*-Bacc-Ed	DoE	X		Ed
PA	RN*, MD, D, U	RN*-BSN-Ed	DoE	X	X	Ed/CE
RI	RN, RN*, HD, MD, D, U	RN*-Bacc-Ed-exp	DoE	X	X	Ed, exp
SC	LPN, RN	LPN, RN	Dist			

(continued)

TABLE 2.1 State Regulations for School Nurse Practice (continued)

State	Authorized to Provide Health Services in Schools	Criteria for Becoming SN	Source of Title	SN Protected Title	SN Mandate	Renewal Requirement
SD	RN, HD, U	RN	Dist		X	
TN	LPN, RN, HD, MD, D, U	LPN, RN	Dist, DoH		X	
TX	LPN, RN, MD, U	RN	Dist	X		
UT	RN, HD, MD, D, U	RN	Dist			
VT	RN*, HD, MD, D	RN*-Ed-exp, RN*-BSN-Ed-exp	DoE	X	X	Ed/CE
VA	LPN, RN, MD, U	RN*-Ed-exp, RN*-BSN-Ed-exp	DoE	X	X	Ed/CE
WA	RN, RN*, PHN, MD	RN*-Ed, RN*-BSN-Ed/exp	DoE	X		Ed/CE, exp
WV	LPN, RN*, HD, MD, D, U	RN*, RN*-BSN-Ed, RN*MSN-NC	DoE	X	X	Ed, MS/age
WI	RN*, RN*, HD, MD, D	RN, RN-BSN-Ed	Dist, DoE	X		Ed/CE if RN*
WY	RN*	RN*- RN-BSN	DoE	X		Ed/CE

Source: Praeger & Zimmerman (2009, p. 469). Reprinted with permission from Sage Publications.

Note: BoN = Board of Nursing; CE = continuing education learning experiences; D = dentist; Dist = local school district; DoE = Department of Education; DoH = Department of Health; Ed = formal or specific course work; exp = experience; HD = health department staff; LPN = licensed practical or vocational nurse; MD = physician or chiropractor; NC = national certification including NBSCN, ANCC, etc.; PHN = public health nurse; RN = registered nurse; RN* = registered nurse credentialed as a school nurse in state; SN = school nurse; U = unlicensed person.

Scope of Practice

Most school nurses work in a public school setting. However, the school nurse may also be employed to work in alternate sites such as residential settings, juvenile justice facilities, or occupational settings. Nurses may also provide services within the community that include after-school events, summer camps, field trips, or sporting events.

Variables

A school nurse's role can differ significantly, depending upon a number of variables. These include the following:

- *Grade level of students*: Prekindergarten, elementary, middle, or high school
- *Size of school*: Small (500 or fewer students), midsized (about 1,000 students), or large (more than 1,000 students)
- *Type of district*: Urban, suburban, or rural
- *Income level of community*: Low, middle, or high
- *Type of school*: Public, parochial, special needs, charter, or residential

Subspecialties

Considering the aforementioned numerous variables, subspecialties have developed that permit a higher level of expertise for a particular group. This specialization fosters even better care and greater understanding of needs. It is logical to expect that the nurse working with preschool-aged handicapped children will have quite a different job than the nurse at an urban high school. Subspecialties might include the following:

- Special needs
- Preschool
- Rural
- Urban
- Suburban
- High school
- Middle school
- Elementary school

THE FUTURE OF SCHOOL NURSING

It is doubtful that our school nurse pioneers ever imagined our profession would grow into what it is today. We can reasonably assume that the need for qualified nurses to care for children will continue to increase for the following reasons:

- Children are spending more time in school through participation in before- and after-school programs, sporting activities, school-sponsored trips, and so on. For many, the school nurse is their only source of medical attention.
- Infant survival has improved and there are more multiple births. These infants frequently have problems at birth and present later in childhood with medical issues in school. The school nurse is needed to ensure their care.
- There are more children with chronic diseases and life-threatening allergies than ever before. School nurses must be available to meet their immediate needs.
- Today's educators now recognize that all children learn from each other. We no longer separate special needs children from their peers, but rather support the placement of children *in the least restrictive environment.* This is the law. School nurses are needed to assess these special children and monitor their medical needs in the academic setting.

3

The School Health Office

After reading the previous chapter, you should have a greater understanding of, and respect for, school nurses and their role in the educational process. Now you are ready to set up the school health office and begin to work in your new home away from home.

The health office, its location, the way it is set up, and how the nurse interacts with students and faculty will establish the school nurse as either a totally insignificant entity or the "heart of the school."

In this chapter, you will learn:

1. Why the health office is an important part of the school
2. How to implement the six steps in the nursing process to assess students' needs
3. When to administer first aid, and how to handle common illnesses and accidents

HEALTH OFFICE LOCATION

The health office should be centrally located and as close as possible to the gym, playground, lunchroom, and any classrooms containing children with life-threatening conditions that could result in a classroom emergency. It must be well lit and ventilated. Air conditioning should be available as needed.

Newer schools were built with these specifications in mind. Many older school buildings were designed appropriately at the time of construction, but as student enrollments grew and more special-services personnel were required by law, the health office may have been moved to a less advantageous location. Making administrators aware of what constitutes a proper health office location may be your first and most difficult task.

Bathroom Facilities

A separate bathroom is essential. Ideally, you should have two sinks: one inside the bathroom, and a clean sink outside the bathroom with an available eye wash station.

FAST FACTS in a NUTSHELL

Consider not providing a lock on the bathroom door. You *must* be able to enter immediately if a student becomes ill while in the bathroom.

Clinical Snapshot

Mrs. S., a long-time faculty member, prefers to use the health office bathroom, which is right next to her classroom, rather than go down the hall to the faculty lounge. She is upset that Darlene, the new school nurse, has had the lock on the bathroom door removed and insists on her privacy, indicating that *the previous nurse allowed a lock*. Darlene explains that this bathroom is for sick children and staff members only. She needs immediate access to anyone who is ill, and Mrs. S. would not want exposure to these germs. Darlene explains that this is her own decision and that it is nonnegotiable.

Health Office Space

A resting place should be available for children who become ill while at school. If space does not permit the separation of a child who is ill from other children, arrange for chairs or a bench to be placed outside the office where students can wait to see you. Leave your door open so that you can monitor them until you have tended to and secluded a child who is ill.

Creating a Warm and Caring Atmosphere

The atmosphere in your office should be warm and welcoming. Permit students and staff to feel that the school health office is a place of refuge. At the same time, avoid allowing any one individual or group to spend excessive amounts of time hanging around. This is not a place for faculty, parent, or student friends to gather and socialize. Your first responsibility is the students' health.

Once your office is arranged properly, you can begin the many other necessary tasks. *See Appendix B for more information regarding assessment tools, first-aid supplies, and other necessary equipment. Appendix C provides a suggested month-by-month calendar of tasks.*

FAST FACTS in a NUTSHELL

Make sure you and your desk are visible from the hall. There are students who will find comfort just knowing you are there in case they need you.

Clinical Snapshot

Lisa, a second grader, has become school phobic. Her parents recently divorced and mom has full custody. Lisa is fearful that, like her dad, mom will also be gone when she comes home from school. School nurse Darlene arranges for Lisa to be left with her in the morning, and Darlene personally walks her to class. Lisa is permitted to pass the health office office several times a day and, seeing Darlene, she is comforted.

Suggestions for Health Office Management

- Invite new students to visit your office when they are not ill. For the lower grades, have the teachers bring their class to you on the first day of school. Older students need assurance as well, so set aside time to meet them and explain your role. Do not miss an opportunity to introduce yourself to new students and parents.

- Be careful whom you allow to use your phone, bathroom, and cot. Once you start permitting these privileges, it is difficult to stop.
- Learn to triage. You will quickly identify the students who are truly ill and those who just want to visit.

THE NURSING PROCESS IN SCHOOL

The nursing process "encompasses all significant actions taken by nurses in providing care to all clients, and forms the foundation for clinical decision making" (American Nurses Association, 1998). Whenever a student enters the health office, the school nurse must follow the appropriate steps of this process.

Six Steps of the School Nursing Process

1. *Assessment:* Note the child's complaint, take vital signs and a history of the complaint, and examine as needed.
2. *Diagnosis:* Formulate a diagnosis, based on the assessment data collected.
3. *Outcome identification:* Identify exactly what you expect to happen with the student.
4. *Planning:* Develop a plan of care or action for the child.
5. *Implementation:* Implement the intervention identified; return the child to class, or exclude him or her from school.
6. *Evaluation:* Evaluate the outcome of the plan; follow up by checking on the student at an appropriate time.

FIRST AID

Regardless of the time of day or evening, when you are in the school building, you are on duty. No other nurse will give you a report at the beginning of your shift, and what you do not finish one day will be waiting for you when you return to the school health office. Every student, staff member, and visitor to the school is your potential patient. You may also be asked to be available for school-sponsored activities, such as sporting events and overnight trips. No two days will be the same, and first aid must be the task you tend to before all others.

Watch the *frequent flyers!* Try to establish an understanding that if a child just wishes to visit he or she can come at an appropriate time; for example, during recess, lunch, or before or after school. The child does not need to invent an illness. This way when he or she is truly ill, you will be less likely to overlook it.

Clinical Snapshot

First-grader Michael comes to School Nurse Darlene complaining that he has a headache. Darlene follows the nursing process to assess him. Michael is pale and appears tired: His temperature is 97.8°F, pulse is 100, blood pressure is 100/60 mmHg. Darlene asks how long he has had the headache and whether he has eaten breakfast (*assessment*). She allows Michael to rest for 10 minutes, noting his body language and how he interacts with other children coming in and out of the office. Michael seems fine (*diagnosis*) after resting, but since he seldom comes to see Darlene, she sends a note to the teacher asking her to observe and refer back if Michael is unable to do his work (*outcome*). Darlene checks on Michael at lunchtime (*plan*), and he tells her his headache is better but she notes he did not finish his lunch. She rechecks his temperature and tells him to let her know if the headache returns (*implementation*). She leaves a message at home alerting Michael's parents of his earlier complaint and poor appetite, and asks that they check him again in the evening (*evaluation*).

This is where your previous experience will come into play. Learning to prioritize tasks is essential; with practice, you will become proficient.

Standing Orders

All school districts should be operating under medical standing orders. These orders are basic guidelines that govern how you are to render first aid. They are based on state codes and are generated by the school nurse and approved, in writing, by the school physician.

Standing orders should be the same throughout a school district and updated annually. If your district does not have standing orders or the procedures are disorganized, work with your district colleagues and school physician to formulate and standardize them. You can solicit samples from other districts and adapt them for your use. Make sure you inform your principal, in writing, that developing standing orders is a mandated task necessary to protect your license and the school district. Share the final product with your principal.

Assessment

All students who seek you out must be appropriately assessed using the nursing process. (For very young students, you may need to speak with parents or teachers to obtain accurate histories.) Most standing orders for rendering first aid are organized into categories: acute illnesses, chronic illnesses, accidents, and behavioral issues. Some common illnesses and basic guidelines to help you properly assess students follow.

Acute Illnesses

Typical acute illnesses of school-aged children include viruses, bacterial infections, rashes, skin lesions, respiratory infections, headaches, and stomachaches.

General Treatment for Acute Illnesses

- Check vital signs; look at the child's throat and ears; listen to breath sounds; feel the abdomen.
- Watch body language; note skin appearance.
- Take the history of the complaint: When did the pain start? Did the child eat breakfast? When did he or she last urinate or have a bowel movement? Was he or she ill during the night? What was he or she doing in class when the pain started?
- Notify a parent. Exclude the child from class if necessary, or tell the parent that you will be checking on the child periodically and that he or she should expect a return call if the child's condition does not improve.
- If these factors are insignificant, keep the child for a short observation period, then allow the child to return to class and recheck the child in an hour or exclude from school.

Chronic Illnesses

Some common chronic illnesses of the school-aged child include allergies, asthma, diabetes, cardiac conditions, tuberculosis, and seizure disorders.

FAST FACTS in a NUTSHELL

It is the goal of the school health program to recognize students' chronic conditions and manage manifestations in school. Unless absolutely necessary, chronically ill children should *not* be excluded because of restrictions secondary to their illnesses. Plans should be in place to control symptoms as they arise so the child can return to class.

Clinical Snapshot

Asthmatic children present a special challenge to school nurses. David, grade 6, needs to take his inhaler before gym class. He is competent in its use and may self-administer. School nurse Darlene wrote an Individualized Healthcare Plan and Emergency Care Plan for his care. Darlene informed David's classroom and physical education teachers of his needs and arranged for him to have a nebulizer with his personal medication available. Darlene is trained in airway management and will not hesitate to summon help if needed.

General Treatment for Chronic Illnesses

Have an Individualized Healthcare Plan (IHP) and an Emergency Care Plan (ECP) in place for each child to address his or her specific condition. The plans should be written by the school nurse in concert with the student, parent(s), physician, teachers, and administrator. They contain the nursing diagnosis, student goals, interventions, evaluation, and specific instructions in the event of an emergency. Plans provided for chronic conditions must include, at a minimum, the following information:

- *Allergies:* the allergen, preventive measures for exposure, and epinephrine autoinjector availability
- *Asthma:* an asthma action plan, medication availability, and nebulizer treatments

- *Diabetes:* snack and exercise schedule, blood glucose testing times, glucagon and other medication needs
- *Cardiac condition:* the nature of the illness and restrictions
- *Tuberculosis:* the medication regimen and follow-up monitoring
- Medication use and oxygen availability

Accidents

Common school accidents include fractures, eye injuries, lacerations, burns, and skull and dental trauma. If severe, do not hesitate to send for an ambulance.

General Treatment for Accidents

- *Fractures:* Apply splints and ice.
- *Eye injuries:* For a foreign body, rinse at the eye station. If the object is not dislodged, loosely cover the eye and refer the person to a physician. For all other eye trauma, refer immediately.
- *Lacerations:* Cleanse, apply a dressing, and refer those with facial and large lacerations to a physician.
- *Burns:* Apply a cool compress; do no break blisters. Call an ambulance if the area involved is large and you suspect a third-degree burn.
- *Head trauma:* Do not move the person; check for bleeding and orientation. Call an ambulance. Head injuries have received increased attention recently. It was once thought that a child's developing brain was more likely to recover fully after an injury because it was flexible and would rewire over time. However, there is now more evidence that deficits manifest years later when the brain is mature and a higher level of reasoning is expected (Brain Injury Association of America, 2004). In all cases involving head trauma, you *must* do the following:
- Document incidents in and out of school on the permanent health record.
- Support you school's policy on sports participation following head trauma. If you feel strongly that it should be tightened, make your concerns known in writing to the school physician and administration.
- Carefully assess every child: Have the child lie down, check pupils, and so on.

- Notify parents even for seemingly minor head injuries.
- *Dental trauma:* Save any teeth in a preservative or the injured person's saliva; refer to a dentist.

===*FAST FACTS in a NUTSHELL*

For situations requiring an ambulance, have the student transported to the closest medical facility. Do *not* wait for parents to arrive at the school. Situations in which an ambulance is definitely needed include:

Suspected or actual anaphylaxis	Head trauma
Airway obstruction or respiratory distress	Large skin burn
Cardiac arrest	Open fracture

Clinical Snapshot

Catherine's mother is a nurse at the regional medical center several towns away. Mom indicates that Catherine is to be taken *only* to her hospital, not the local one closest to the school. School nurse Darlene discusses this in advance and clarifies with her that all emergencies must be treated as such and transferred to the *closest facility*. Once there, parents can sign out and transfer their child wherever they wish.

Behavioral Issues

Behavioral issues can include school phobia, tantrums, depression, and anxiety disorders. Frequently, the school nurse becomes involved in helping students who are experiencing separation issues or emotional problems. Beware of the frequent visitor. It is easy to miss a true illness in a child who sees you every day with minor complaints.

General Treatment for Behavioral Issues

- Communicate closely with the student, parent(s), and teachers.
- Develop a plan.
- Refer to specific professional help and remain available.

ROLE OF SCHOOL NURSES IN RENDERING FIRST AID

- *You* make the assessment. Do not be influenced by teachers or parents.
- Assess every child who enters your office. Remain calm and confident.
- Discourage students, parents, and colleagues from coming to school for you to diagnose when they are ill. You are not a physician.
- If you are uncertain whether a child should be sent home or to the hospital in an ambulance, call 911. *Always err on the side of caution.*
- Learn to triage and remain current on all first-aid procedures.
- Prominently display in your office and on your phone the emergency numbers and names of other people in your school who are certified in cardiopulmonary resuscitation and use of an automated external defibrillator.
- Call the child's parent(s) for even minor issues. This allows the parent(s) to decide whether to ignore the problem, come into school immediately to evaluate the child themselves, or deal with a situation at home.
- When asked for a physician referral, offer the names of several local doctors. Allow parents to choose for themselves.
- Have accurate, updated emergency contact information available for every child and adult in your building.

4

The Big Three: Immunizations, Screenings, and Medications

Monitoring immunizations, performing screenings, and administering medications are three of the major areas in school nursing practice for which we are totally responsible. We are the gatekeepers for maintaining school compliance for all immunizations; detecting, referring, and following up on vision, hearing, height, weight, blood pressure, and scoliosis through mass screenings; and giving medications so students can remain in school and function at their highest level of wellness.

The big three represent our overwhelming responsibility to children, our employers, and our profession.

In this chapter, you will learn:

1. The school nurse's responsibility in immunization monitoring
2. Basic elements of the screening process
3. General guidelines for administering medications

IMMUNIZATIONS

The control of communicable diseases was one of the original reasons for placing nurses in school settings and remains a major responsibility of school nurses today. Administrators depend on school nurses to uphold health regulations and to keep them informed of any deficiencies.

FAST FACTS in a NUTSHELL

Every state has immunization requirements for children who attend school. It is imperative that you know your state and district policies regarding immunization requirements, the parental rights of refusal, and the reportable infectious diseases.

Clinical Snapshot

David recently transferred into the school where Samantha is the nurse. Records from his previous, out-of-state school indicate that he is in full compliance with all required immunizations. However, your state requires additional immunizations. The different policy must be explained to the parents and David should be permitted to attend school while receiving the remaining required immunizations.

Many parents question the safety of the numerous vaccines required today and mistrust or resist government requirements. These parents have a right to express their concerns to you. However, if a large number of parents refuse immunizations for their children, preventable diseases will reemerge and cause illnesses and deaths, as they have in the past. For the overall health of all students, it is imperative that all be fully immunized according to state public health requirements. The recommended immunizations for children from birth through 6 years of age and 7 through 18 years of age are provided in Appendix D.

Generally, you may accept immunization documentation from the following sources:

- A private physician: assigned certificate, prescription, or note with letterhead
- A public health department: official record
- A previous school: official school or child care records

Each entry must contain the complete date (month, day, and year).

Healthy People 2020 Objectives
Immunization and Infectious Diseases, 19
Increase the number of states collecting kindergarten vaccine coverage data according to the CDC minimum standards from 13 in 2009 to 51 (including the District of Columbia).

FAST FACTS in a NUTSHELL

Be aware that many countries list the day first, then the month and year. For example, an immunization given in the United States on December 2, 2002, would be recorded as 12/2/2002; the same date could be recorded internationally as 02/12/2002.

Clinical Snapshot

School nurse Samantha had to translate the recorded birth date for a student from the United Kingdom and then recheck all the dates of the immunizations to make sure vaccines were given at the appropriate ages and intervals according to her state's laws.

You may encounter parents who have not had their children immunized for a variety of reasons, including strong religious or philosophical beliefs, fear, indifference, or ignorance. Parents are not forced to make a decision regarding immunization until their children enter school and the governing laws demand compliance before admission. This can be a difficult situation. Be sympathetic, yet firm, and stress that you are implementing a state law.

Contraindications for Immunizations

Medical

It is not required to give a child any immunization that is medically contraindicated. Requests for exemption must state the reason and the period of time for which immunization is to be withheld, and must be signed by a physician.

Religious

If a required immunization conflicts with the student's religious beliefs or practices, the parents must request the exemption in writing. The document must state how the vaccine conflicts with the religious beliefs or practices. A copy of the document should be forwarded to your administrator for legal review. This is *not* the same as a philosophical, moral, or conscientious exemption.

Provisional

A child may be allowed to attend school after he or she has received an initial dose of the required immunization and is in the process of completing the series. Parents must keep you updated as immunizations are given.

Role of School Nurses in Meeting Immunization Requirements

- Strongly recommend that all health information be submitted *before* children enter school. Get administrative support to exclude those who are noncompliant.
- Review any new student's information: registration form, health history, physical examination, immunizations received, previous school records, emergency card, and so on.
- Document dates on each permanent health record and review annually, noting any recent changes in requirements.
- Refer back to the physician or clinic for deficiencies.
- Recheck *all* students' immunizations for deficiencies at least annually.
- Review and update students' records with medical, religious, and provisional status.
- Know your state's immunization regulations. File the immunization status report as required in your state and allow local or state officials access to your files for the purposes of audit or survey.
- Be cautious with noncompliant parents. Refer back to private physicians for reassurances as to safety.

Until a child reaches the age when he or she is required by law to attend school, parents can choose not to immunize their child. If that is the case, you will be the first one to confront the parent with the law.

Clinical Snapshot

Mr. and Mrs. K. register their twin boys in May for kindergarten. School nurse Samantha notes that neither has received any immunizations. Both parents are adamant that their children *not* receive immunizations or any foreign substance in their bodies. Samantha states that although she believes in the importance of protecting children from disease, she respects their rights as parents. She informs the parents that she is serving as an agent of the board of education and must act according to the laws of the state and district. She agrees to work with them and provide steps they must take to resolve the issue. She explains that they can seek a medical or religious exemption, and the process involved. She remains nonjudgmental and forwards all information to the principal for the school attorney for review.

SCREENINGS

Screenings are considered the secondary level of prevention. The goal is early detection and prompt treatment of deficiencies *before* they become health problems. When children are screened, those with no obvious problem are separated from those who need to be seen by a physician.

Role of School Nurses in the Screening Process

- Know the district and state laws relevant to screening in the school setting.
- Have all equipment calibrated and in good working condition; know how to use it.
- Obtain necessary written permission from parents.
- Know the grade levels, previous referrals, and special students that must be screened yearly.
- Seek cooperation from staff to arrange for students to be screened at mutually convenient times.

FAST FACTS in a NUTSHELL

You may choose to do all your screenings individually or allot a certain amount of time per student and do all the screenings at once. Do what works best for you and is the least disruptive for the students and teachers. States vary significantly in the number and types of required health screenings.

Clinical Snapshot

School nurse Samantha schedules each child for a 10-minute block of time when performing mandated screenings. She sends for three students at a time, has them bring material to read while waiting, and performs all screenings—vision, hearing, height, weight, blood pressure, and scoliosis—during this visit. Samantha enjoys this time with each child and the opportunity to talk with them individually.

Samantha's colleagues prefer to do each screening separately. They feel this provides an opportunity to see every student at least several times throughout the school year, and not just those who are *frequent flyers*.

- Using the guidelines recommended by your school physician, make referrals after you have checked several times or immediately if you find a defect that is profound.
- Document findings on worksheets; transfer them to the permanent record.
- Follow up on all referrals to see that care is rendered.
- Let parents know that if they do not hear from you, they may assume their child passed the screening.
- Recheck all students who fail the initial screening at least once before sending out a referral.

FAST FACTS in a NUTSHELL

Be sensitive to the child's right to privacy. Do *not* announce the child's weight or any other information for others to hear.

Clinical Snapshot

Samantha makes certain that students cannot see the scale numbers and refuses to tell any child what they weigh while she is screening them. She tells students to see her after school if they wish to know the numbers.

Ask your administrator to allow you to screen without inter-ruptions. Request that the principal designate someone to handle nonurgent issues.

Clinical Snapshot

Samantha informed the office secretary and principal of the times she and the classroom teachers had agreed upon for screenings. She was interrupted three times during the first 30 minutes to attend to a child with an upset stomach, a student who wanted to use the phone to call home for sneakers, and a child with a nosebleed that had stopped by the time Samantha got to him. Samantha had to explain the importance of this time for proper assessment and asked that she should only be disturbed for an *emergency*. Samantha then defined an *emergency*.

If the interruptions continue, Samantha should request a substitute to cover her office while she is screening students.

Typical School Screenings for All Students

Blood pressure	Height, weight, body mass index
Dental	Scoliosis
Drug	Tuberculosis
Hearing	Vision

Consider planning your screenings according to the season. The few minutes you save in attending to each child add up.

Clinical Snapshot

Samantha schedules height and weight screenings at the beginning of the school year so she can see and talk with every student and identify immediate problems. She tries to complete all the hearing screenings before the temperature drops and the cold season begins, knowing that head congestion will interfere with a reliable result. Samantha holds off on blood pressure screening until the spring, when children are more likely to wear short sleeves; this allows for quicker cuff placement.

MEDICATIONS

Administration of medications, both prescribed and over-the-counter, is an area of high risk and can be extremely difficult for the school nurse. Because of the large number of students with chronic health conditions and disabilities, often there is no choice but to medicate while at school. The nurse has an obligation to ensure that the procedure for safe dispensing is closely followed. Accept medications only in original containers.

Most school policies demand an annual written order from a physician or advanced practice nurse and a signed parental consent to dispense medications. Standardized forms for this purpose are usually available for parents and physicians to use.

People Authorized to Give Medication in School

School policies usually permit only the following people to dispense medications:

- The school physician
- A certified or noncertified nurse employed by the district
- A substitute school nurse employed by the district
- A student's parent or guardian
- A student who is approved to self-administer in certain life-threatening conditions, such as anaphylaxis or asthma.
- School employees trained and delegated to administer medication in emergencies

FAST FACTS in a NUTSHELL

Do not make exceptions for *anyone* regarding routine medication administration. Stick to the official policy, for your protection and that of the district.

◉ Clinical Snapshot

School nurse Samantha worked for years in a hospital setting. She knew of numerous nurses who had made medication errors. Typically, the first reported error was handled by a warning. If a second occurred, the nurse would be sent for a remedial lesson on medication administration. The third error would result in termination. Schools are quite different. That first error could mean your job. Be cautious and stick to district policy.

Epinephrine, Glucagon, and Diastat Administration and Delegate Training

Schools are required to have policies in place to deal with anaphylactic reactions for diagnosed and undiagnosed children with life-threatening allergies. It is your responsibility to have the medication available and to train any delegates to recognize symptoms and to use the proper technique to administer the injection.

Many states also have regulations permitting glucagon or Diastat administration by noncertified personnel. You will be responsible for delegate training for these individuals, as well.

Field Trips

If a child requires medication at any school-sponsored event, nursing coverage may be required. A policy must be in place and a substitute nurse hired to attend the event.

Types of Medications Given at School

Behavior Modification

Today, many of these drugs are given once a day at home. You may offer to keep one dose available in case a parent calls to tell you that a dose was missed at home. You must still have an order from the physician and written parental consent.

Antibiotics

Unless written in a health care plan, administer only if the medication is ordered three or four times a day.

Emergencies

- Asthma: oral inhalers, nebulizers
- Epinephrine, Benadryl, Glucagon, Diastat

There are numerous gray areas in the practice of school nursing. Do not hesitate to send the ill child home, call an ambulance, or uphold your medication policy. This may mean that you are not loved by everyone but that is okay.

Clinical Snapshot

Samantha replaced a beloved school nurse who had worked in the same location for 25 years. Samantha constantly meets resistance to any change she attempts. Samantha will need to learn to choose her battles, compromise when she can, and be forceful when necessary in hopes that in time she will be appreciated for the contribution she makes to the school.

ROLE OF SCHOOL NURSES IN MEDICATION ADMINISTRATION

- Know your district policy on medications and follow it exactly. If you disagree with how it is written, get clarification before it becomes an issue.
- Avoid giving medications in school whenever possible. Herbal remedies, food supplements, and medications ordered once or twice a day can be taken at home.
- It is preferable for the first and second doses of antibiotics be given at home in case of a reaction.
- Carefully document the medication given for each student.
- Have physicians' orders and signed parental consents updated yearly.
- Permit students to self-administer according to state regulations and school policy.
- Train delegates to administer emergency medications as permitted by state regulations and school policy.

PART

II

Health Appraisal

Health Promotion and Disease Prevention

5

Student Health Assessments

Starting sometime in early May, excitement commences as parents initiate the "school crusade" on behalf of their children. They insist on certain teachers and arrangements for the upcoming fall classes. Then comes the flood of July advertisements for school clothes, sneakers, backpacks, and other paraphernalia that parents purchase to ensure that their children have the essential tools for success in school.

Yet these same conscientious parents may never consider scheduling routine health examinations for their children. They may give no thought to whether their children are physically and emotionally ready for school and capable of fully participating in the sports program. This is where the school nurse steps in.

In this chapter, you will learn:

1. Why periodic health assessments are essential to learning, and when the most appropriate times are to make them
2. Major reasons for poor school attendance
3. The history, and the pros and cons, of school-based clinics

STUDENT HEALTH ASSESSMENTS

Physical examinations for schoolchildren began as far back as 1920. Their purpose was to identify children with "defects" (Wold, 1981), with the rationale that no student's learning potential should be compromised by a remediable physical disability and that every student should be able to participate fully in all school activities and be free of communicable diseases. The examinations were done at school or by private physicians.

Critics argued that examinations performed at school were too costly and superficial; without parental input, there could be no complete detection of health problems.

Beginning around 1950, most required examinations were performed by private physicians in their offices. These examinations were more comprehensive than those that had been performed at school but proved to be costly in time and money for the parents. Often, students were noncompliant and districts were left with the difficult decision of whether such children should be excluded from school, physical education class, or sports.

FAST FACTS in a NUTSHELL

Today, school examinations are referred to as health assessments because subjective and objective information must be gathered and interpreted by the health professional. The entire body, from head to toe, is considered, as is a child's emotional wellness.

Clinical Snapshot

School nurse Joan frequently checks with the parents of children she knows have emotional issues. If she is aware that a student has been absent for a prolonged period or is suffering from depression, she initiates a call giving a heads up about any problem and inquires how the student is doing at home.

All schools require physical assessments according to state law or local district policy. They may vary in frequency and depth. Most districts offer assessments in school or will help to arrange free clinic visits for students. Assessments are performed by physicians or advanced practice nurses.

Types of Assessments

School nurses are concerned with two types of assessments: routine wellness and athletic assessments.

Routine Assessments

Routine assessments can be required of students:

- Upon entrance to school within a specified period of time (usually 1 year)
- During the early childhood years (grades K–3)
- During preadolescence (grades 4–6)
- Upon reaching adolescence (grades 7–12)
- When referred for Child Study Team evaluation
- When applying for work permits
- When suspected of drug abuse

A routine assessment must note any health problems and state clearly whether the student may or may not participate in physical education classes. It must identify any physical education restrictions, and, if it is conducted at school, parental consent must be obtained in writing. A physician-signed, standardized form is commonly used.

Athletic Assessments

Most school districts now have specific procedures and forms for participation in athletics. Assessments and questionnaires usually must be completed within a certain time frame before a sport begins. An athletic assessment includes, at minimum, the following components:

- A detailed health history, signed by the parent or guardian, which covers previous injuries, surgeries, loss of consciousness, and so on
- A comprehensive physical examination, including blood and urine analysis
- A statement from the examining physician permitting the student to participate
- Provisions for updates throughout the school year for other sports
- Written permission from the parent for the student to be examined and participate in the sport
- School-physician approval for all private-physician clearances

Role of School Nurses in Assessments

- Know, understand, and implement the policies and procedures for the district.
- Scrutinize physical examination reports, noting any restrictions. Upon a physician's order or for any student not cleared in writing, exclude the student from participation in physical education classes and athletic competitions.
- Provide physical education teachers and coaches with a list of students who may not participate.
- Carefully document the results of all assessments on the permanent health record.
- If an assessment is done in school, provide necessary equipment and assistance.
- Advocate for children. If you believe that participation in athletics is not in a child's best interest, put it in writing.

ATTENDANCE

According to law, every child is entitled to a free public education. To get such an education, a student must be well enough to learn and attend school consistently.

FAST FACTS in a NUTSHELL

Every child should be accounted for every day. This does not mean that nurses, themselves, need to make calls to check on absences. This should be the responsibility of office staff. The school nurse must be in touch with seriously ill children and follow up with those who are sent home.

Clinical Snapshot

As did her predecessor, school nurse Joan spends almost the entire morning handling attendance problems. However, Joan's job now also includes teaching two classes of health education a day and she is becoming increasingly frustrated. She hates leaving her office when the attendance is incomplete and resents tracking down parents who do not call in. When she spoke with the principal, he said there was no one else to perform this clerical task. Nonetheless, Joan began to document the hours spent on attendance and once the waste of professional time was itemized, the principal and Joan reached a compromise. The secretary would handle routine absences and Joan would follow up on serious illnesses and accidents.

- Chronic health conditions (asthma, cancer, etc.)
- Poverty
- Frequent family moves
- Unrest at home
- Feelings of isolation or not being connected with school
- Gaps in learning, especially in lower grades that provide the foundation for math and reading

Children with prolonged and frequent absences are at risk for failure in school. These children may choose to drop out altogether. Students are much more likely to succeed in school when they attend consistently. In addition, school budgets may suffer when absentee rates are high. State and federal funds may be awarded to schools that have low absentee rates, providing more money for essential classroom needs.

FAST FACTS in a NUTSHELL

All too often, children who are homeschooled or placed out of the district fall through the cracks. Remember, these are still your students. Your district is paying for a service in another school. The greater the number of people who monitor the child, the safer he or she will be. You have a place in this process, especially if the placement is for a medical need. Maintain contact with the parents or the school nurse in the out-of-district school(s), or both.

Clinical Snapshot

Mrs. K. has three children. The youngest, Amy, has special needs that require placement in a regional special education program. On a day when the rest of the staff is attending a math inservice program, school nurse Joan requests and receives permission to visit Mrs. K's child. Joan spends time in the classroom talking with Amy and her teacher. She then stops in to see the school nurse. Joan is more than pleased with the care Amy is receiving and tells Mrs. K. Joan also suggests to the Child Study Team that Amy be permitted to join her grade-level peers for special events in her school. Mrs. K is appreciative and thanks her for not forgetting her child and for fostering inclusion.

Role of School Nurses in Monitoring Attendance

- Know your students, why they are not in school, and, if possible, try to remedy the problem.
- Monitor students who are frequently tardy or absent.
- Review and enforce the school policy on absenteeism.
- Control contagious diseases as much as possible: Exclude ill students from school, discourage acutely ill students from returning to school too quickly, and send notices home informing parents of any widespread illnesses.
- Encourage healthful habits: frequent hand washing, cleanliness, room ventilation, adequate rest and exercise, and proper nutrition. Be proactive in keeping your students healthy.
- Work to identify the true cause of absenteeism before a child is penalized unfairly.

Healthy People 2020 Objectives

Access to Health Services, 5.2

Increase the proportion of children and youth aged 17 years and under who have a specific source of ongoing care from 94.3 in 2008 to 100%.

SCHOOL-BASED CLINICS

In the mid-1960s, during President Johnson's War on Poverty, it was noted that poor children in the United States were medically underserved. The establishment of Medicaid in 1965 increased the focus on the plight of low-income families. Because children were required to spend many hours a day at school, it was felt that schools were the logical place to provide the care offered by Medicaid. The rationale was as follows:

- Schools were more convenient and comfortable for students, especially in dealing with mental health issues. Health education could be directly targeted to those in need (Brodeurk, 2002).
- Many families had inadequate or no health insurance, leaving children with few options for medical treatment.
- Schools dealt with many medically fragile students. On-site care was thought to be most beneficial.

Opponents of school-based clinics argued the following points:

- Children should not be given information about birth control at the clinics. Some felt that this would do little to affect risky sexual behavior.
- Funding was difficult. Multiple sources of income were necessary and not always forthcoming.

In 1986, the Robert Wood Johnson Foundation launched an adolescent health care program. It awarded grants up to $600,000 each to public and private schools in poor, overcrowded urban areas to set up adolescent health care centers. One of the grant criteria was that the staff of these clinics were to cooperate with school nurses, teachers, coaches, counselors, and school principals and their staff.

The clinics were required to provide a comprehensive range of services, including the following:

- Treatment for common illnesses and minor injuries
- Referrals and follow-up for serious illnesses and emergencies
- On-site care and consultations, and follow-up for pregnancies
- Counseling and referrals for drug and alcohol abuse, sexual abuse, and risks of suicide
- On-site care and referrals for sexually transmitted diseases
- Sports and employment physicals
- Immunizations

It is estimated that there are now more than 1,900 school-based health clinics in the United States. Serving thousands of students, they are staffed with nurse practitioners and part-time physicians.

═══════════════════════ *FAST FACTS in a NUTSHELL*

Providing all students with appropriate health care is a challenge. Suspect financial difficulties when medical forms are not returned. Assist families to find services and follow through until their needs are met.

Clinical Snapshot

School nurse Joan is well aware of the families in her district that have low income levels and receive health care through the clinic of the local hospital. She does not always know of the family going through temporary tough times. She should suspect there is a financial problem when a parent is compliant with all school health requirements except those that cost money.

ROLE OF SCHOOL NURSES IN SCHOOL-BASED CLINICS

- Establish open lines of communication between the school health office and the local clinic. Remember, you both have the same goals.
- Refer students as needed.
- Remain diligent in protecting students' rights and privacy.
- If you are in a district where students' health needs are not being met, seek a remedy. Explore the possibility of a school-based clinic.

6

Health Education

It has long been recognized that the most influential factor in a child's ability to learn is the teacher(s). Health, more than any other discipline, must be taught by well-qualified professionals who know the content and are comfortable with it. When that teacher has extensive, practical knowledge in the field and has already demonstrated a strong commitment to students, it is definitely a winning combination.

The school nurse is the perfect health educator; he or she has a strong medical background, is current on health issues, and is deeply devoted to children. With one foot in nursing and the other in education, the school nurse is the ideal person to identify, teach, and demonstrate healthful habits.

Health education is at the very core of the thrust toward primary prevention. Nurses teach instinctively every day of their professional lives, sometimes before a large group but more often informally, with the same good outcome.

In this chapter, you will learn:

1. The definition of health education and its function as a separate discipline
2. Risk factors for young people
3. The national standards for health education

4. The content of health education
5. How to teach health
6. Obstacles to teaching health education

HEALTH EDUCATION

Definition

Health education is the totality of experiences that influence knowledge of, and attitudes toward, health. It should be meaningful to the learners, motivate them to maintain and improve their health, and provide them with the knowledge and skills they need in order to be healthy for a lifetime.

Health education has functioned as a separate discipline for a number of decades. However, it is still considered a relatively new discipline and struggles for a sense of identity (Gilbert, 2000, p. 5). For health learning to have taken place, there must be a positive change in behavior.

Comprehensive Health Education

Health education works. Hundreds of studies have evaluated health education and concluded that it is effective in reducing the number of teenage pregnancies, decreasing smoking rates among young people, and preventing the adoption of many high-risk behaviors (Summerfield, 1998).

A sequential comprehensive program rather than sporadic health lectures serves best to introduce healthful lifestyle habits; therefore, we should seek to offer comprehensive health education in our schools. A school health education curriculum is an organized, sequential kindergarten-through-grade-12 plan for teaching students and helping them develop life skills that will improve their health, prevent diseases, and reduce health-related risk behaviors (Meeks, Heit & Page, 2009, p. 20).

It is not enough to offer health education periodically, as issues arise. Health should be taught, as other disciplines, by building concepts and skills in a sequential, organized fashion.

Clinical Snapshot

Jennifer, a school nurse and health teacher, was invited into a fifth grade class to discuss the dangers of smoking. When she began explaining how cigarette residue interferes with the exchange of air in the aveoli, she realized the students had no knowledge of the anatomy of the lungs. Had this information been included in earlier lessons, a brief review would have been all that was required for the fifth graders.

Comprehensive health education in the classroom:

- Addresses the physical, mental, emotional, and social dimensions of health
- Develops health knowledge, attitudes, and skills
- Is tailored to each age level
- Is designed to motivate and assist students to maintain and improve their health and prevent disease

Healthy People 2020 Objectives

Early and Middle Childhood, 4.3

Increase the proportion of schools that require cumulative instruction in health education that meet the U.S. National Health Education Standards for elementary, middle, and high schools:

Elementary—from 7.5% in 2006 to 11.5%

Middle—from 10.3% in 2006 to 14.3%

High—from 6.5% in 2006 to 10.5%

RISK FACTORS FOR YOUNG PEOPLE

The Centers for Disease Control and Prevention (CDC) have identified six categories of priority health-risk behaviors among youth and young adults:

1. Behaviors that contribute to unintentional injuries and violence (accidents, suicide, etc.)
2. Tobacco use
3. Alcohol and drug use
4. Sexual behaviors that contribute to unintended pregnancy and sexually transmitted diseases
5. Unhealthful dietary behaviors
6. Physical inactivity

Results from the *2009 National Youth Risk Behavior Surveillance Report* indicate that many high school students engage in behaviors that increase their likelihood for the leading causes of death among persons aged 10 to 24 years in the United States. The report summarizes results from the 2009 national survey, which included 42 state surveys and 20 local surveys of students in grades 9 to 12:

- 28.3% had ridden in a car driven by someone who had been drinking alcohol
- 19.5% had smoked cigarettes
- 41.8% had drunk alcohol within 30 days of taking the survey
- 34.2% were sexually active and 38.9% did not use a condom during their last sexual encounter
- 77.7% did not eat recommended amounts of fruit and vegetables
- 81.6% were not physically active for at least 60 minutes every day
- 12% were obese (Centers for Disease Control and Prevention, 2010).

THE NATIONAL HEALTH EDUCATION STANDARDS

To address the above-mentioned concerns, standards were developed to help states and local districts meet the needs of students. These standards provide health educators with a blueprint for local district curriculum development, instruction, and assessment that reflect the latest research-based data.

The national health education standards are written to be deliberately vague, allowing teachers to adapt them to the needs of their individual classes and students.

🔘 Clinical Snapshot

Jennifer has just completed screenings in height and weight and calculating body mass indexes for students. She notes that 30% of the eighth grade class is obese. Before developing her lessons, she must identify the common cause and direct her lessons accordingly. Her focus should be on current diet and exercise habits and the long-term effects on health.

In 2006, the Joint Committee on Health Education Standards established the following guidelines for health education:

- Specify what students should know.
- Specify what students should be able to do.
- Knowledge and skills involved are essential to the development of health literacy.
- Skills include communication, reasoning, and investigating.

The National Health Education Standards include the following:

Standard 1	Students will comprehend concepts related to health promotion and disease prevention to enhance health.
Standard 2	Students will analyze the influence of family, peers, culture, media, technology, and other factors on health behaviors.
Standard 3	Students will demonstrate the ability to access valid information and products and services to enhance health.
Standard 4	Students will demonstrate the ability to use interpersonal communication skills to enhance health and avoid or reduce health risks.
Standard 5	Students will demonstrate the ability to use decision-making skills to enhance health.

(continued)

Standard 6	Students will demonstrate the ability to use goal-setting skills to enhance health.
Standard 7	Students will demonstrate the ability to practice health-enhancing behaviors and avoid or reduce risks.
Standard 8	Students will demonstrate the ability to advocate for personal, family, and community health (Centers for Disease Control and Prevention, 2013a).

Needs Assessment

Using these national standards as a guide, states and local districts work to address the specific needs of their students and develop further core standards to reference when planning health curricula. From these curricula, the units of instruction are developed and specific lesson plans are designed.

State Curriculum Content Standards

There are state curriculum standards for all disciplines, including health and physical education. These standards are revised at least every 5 years. They provide consistency throughout each state; help improve student learning; form the foundation for assessment, curriculum development, and instruction; and serve as a guide for writing lesson plans.

As an example of these standards, the New Jersey Core Curriculum Content Standards for Health are as follows:

- All students will acquire health promotion concepts and skills to support a healthy, active lifestyle.
- All students will develop and use personal and interpersonal skills to support a healthy, active lifestyle.
- All students will acquire knowledge about alcohol, tobacco, other drugs, and medicines and apply these concepts to support a healthy, active lifestyle.
- All students will acquire knowledge about the physical, emotional, and social aspects of human relationships and sexuality and apply these concepts to support a healthy, active lifestyle (New Jersey Department of Education, 2014)

School health education programs should be based on local needs—the health behaviors and problems within the school population. According to the American School Health Association (1994), there are 10 general areas to address:

1. Community health
2. Consumer health
3. Environmental health
4. Personal health and fitness
5. Family life education
6. Nutrition and healthy eating
7. Disease prevention and control
8. Safety and injury prevention
9. Prevention of substance use and abuse (alcohol, tobacco, drugs)
10. Growth and development

FAST FACTS in a NUTSHELL

As you develop your units and lessons, remember that learning will not take place unless the topic is relevant to the needs of the learner. Know your students and plan accordingly.

Clinical Snapshot

School nurse Jennifer spent hours developing a comprehensive unit on the different food groups for her 10th grade classes. She is disheartened when students show no interest and are rude and inattentive. In hindsight, Jennifer realizes that this is a boring, repetitive topic for this age group. More relevant topics for high school students would be eating disorders or fad diets.

Health Literacy

An important concept underlying health education is health literacy. This includes having a sound knowledge base so that when students complete their health education in school they can go forward capable of making sound health decisions in their lives.

We want them to think critically, have good communication skills, and be contributing members of society.

TEACHING HEALTH

Steps for Teaching Health

- Identify general health-risk factors of the population as a whole.
- Reference the national and state standards.
- Consider the topics listed for that month by the National Health Observances (see Appendix E).
- Assess your students' needs.
- Develop the curriculum with assistance from colleagues and the administration. Have the curriculum approved by the principal, and present it at an open board meeting where parents can have input.
- Plan the unit of instruction to cover each content area.
- Develop the lesson plan in a way that is specific to the needs of your students.
- Implement the lesson plan.
- Evaluate the lesson plan and revise it as often as needed to accommodate the changing needs of students.
- Keep parents informed, especially when teaching issues that are controversial or involve sexuality.

Inservice Education for Staff Members

According to state and district policy, teachers and other school staff members must receive instruction on a number of health topics on a yearly or biennial basis. This provides an excellent opportunity for school nurses to demonstrate their teaching skills and establish themselves as health educators.

Procedure for Providing Inservice Education for Staff Members

- Identify topics in your policy and procedure book for which education is required (child abuse, bloodborne pathogens, suicide, anaphylaxis, safety, etc.)
- Write a topic agenda and have it approved by the school administration.

- Arrange an appropriate time and place for inservice education.
- Develop a PowerPoint or overhead-transparency presentation.
- Have the staff complete an evaluation of your program.
- Award inservice credit if it is given in your district.

Role of School Nurses in Health Education

- Be a role model for healthful habits.
- Make resources available to teachers and students.
- Help plan the health curriculum.
- Teach one-on-one, to small groups, or in the classroom.
- Serve as a health consultant to students and colleagues.
- Stay current on health issues.
- Do not allow yourself to become so overwhelmed with procedural tasks and first aid that you have no time to teach, in and out of the classroom.
- Offer additional staff inservice education as issues arise.

OBSTACLES TO CLASSROOM HEALTH TEACHING

Perceived Poor Classroom Management Skills

The most logical approach here is to seek assistance from the experienced master teachers in your school or district. Observe them teaching and then have them critique your lessons. Follow their examples and ask for suggestions.

Lack of Time to Prepare and Implement Lessons

If you have a teaching schedule or the same contract as your colleagues, you are entitled to preparation time in your schedule. Speak to your administrator or, if necessary, your union representative.

Concern Over Handling Sensitive Issues

Know your curriculum. If it has been board approved and parents have been notified of the content, you may answer questions and deal with sensitive issues in an age-appropriate manner. Notify parents when sensitive sexual topics are planned and allow them the opportunity to review the lesson content and, if they wish, exclude their children.

Frustrations With Constant Interruptions or Lack of Health Office Coverage

Clarify with the school administration who will make student assessments or decisions, and decide whether to interrupt your class, when you are teaching. Define to that person what constitutes a *true* emergency, and give specific instructions about how nonurgent problems are to be handled until you finish teaching.

Low Priority Given to Health Education Compared With Other Disciplines

Students are given standardized tests for math, reading, science, and other content areas. These scores are made public, and schools tend to focus time and energy on raising their students' scores so that they are seen in a favorable light by parents and other districts. Health education is seldom measured with a standardized test that is made public.

School nurses need to remind all involved of the importance of health education and the need for students to be well enough to learn. The true test of this goal is students' ability to make good lifestyle choices. This is impossible to measure in the short term.

Take it upon yourself to initiate opportunities to demonstrate your teaching skills. Do not become so bogged down with procedural tasks that administrators and colleagues forget that you are a competent nurse *and* teacher. Sometimes you need to escape from your office to see the bigger picture.

Clinical Snapshot

School nurse Jennifer hates lunchtime recess. There usually is standing room only in the school health office because of numerous playground injuries. Frustrated, she decides to go outside and observe what is going on. She notes that supervision is inadequate and some playground practices are unsafe. Jennifer speaks with the principal and physical education teacher and organizes a safety inservice program on playground use for the staff and lunch aides. Children playing recklessly are made to sit for a designated time. Fewer injuries now occur, and Jennifer has more time to focus on the unavoidable injuries.

PART

III

Professional Issues

Professional Issues

7

Documentation

"If it was not documented, it was not done." These might have been among the first words you heard when you started your nursing studies. Today the words remain true and carry even greater significance in school health. Remember, a school nurse works alone. If you do not document appropriately, no one else will.

It is no secret that we are living in litigious times. Legal actions against school boards of education are far too common, and the great majority of these actions are centered on the delivery of health care. What you do for children is certainly important; however, how you document your actions is just as important. You must always be able to provide written evidence that you acted correctly.

In this chapter, you will learn:

1. Concerns about documentation
2. Information required for students' individual health folders
3. Assessment information needed for daily log entries
4. How to maintain emergency health cards
5. How to complete some administrative reports required in your state and district

DOCUMENTATION CONCERNS

School nurses face decisions every day regarding health information: how much should be written in files, where they should be stored, and who should be permitted to see these files. Often, unauthorized personnel have access to private data.

Recordkeeping tasks are endless and time consuming. They keep school nurses from spending valuable time directly with our students. We grudgingly do it, and far too frequently, we omit valuable information. Each school district has some variation as to the types of forms used for documentation, but a number of documents are required by all districts.

INDIVIDUAL HEALTH FOLDERS

Every student must have his or her own folder, containing, at a minimum, the following documents:

- A permanent, cumulative health form that includes:
  - The student's birth date
  - The parents' names, address(es), and phone numbers
  - Screening data
  - A record of immunizations
  - Growth and development information
  - Disease history
  - Blood pressure
  - Tuberculosis testing results
  - Lead testing results
  - Dental examination data
  - A nurses' notes section containing the date of enrollment, any transfers, and any further significant health information
- Health information taken from initial registration
- Previous school health records
- An individual student log sheet
- An immunization record
- An individual medication record
- Referrals and follow-ups
- Copies of accident or incident reports
- Any correspondence from parents, physicians, teachers, and so on
- A report of physical examinations

- Notes about any exclusions from physical education classes or school
- Your personal notes, which are not included on the permanent record

=======================================*FAST FACTS in a NUTSHELL*

An individual health folder is a legal document. All entries should be made in ink, with the exception of the student's address and phone numbers. Errors should be bracketed and initialed. Do not erase or white out anything that has been written.

Clinical Snapshot

Adriana, the certified school nurse, is paid a stipend to come to school in early August. She personally reviews incoming students' health records. Parents must sign consents for her to receive the information. Adriana insists on this background information from sending districts. Sometimes her forms are more inclusive than theirs and further information is needed. Preparing in August gives her time to review information before the children enter school in September.

Role of School Nurses in Documentation in Individual Health Folders

- Gather and carefully review all available medical information for the incoming student. Note any restrictions, major illnesses, operations, and so on. If the student is transferring into your school, send for the permanent health record from the previous school, note when the student was admitted to your school in the nurses' notes section, and continue adding information as needed.
- List all deficiencies and notify parents of these, along with a deadline for any examination, referral, or immunization required.
- Follow up on all deficiencies and referrals. Inform the administration of those who are noncompliant.

- If this is the first school for the student, or if the health records are unobtainable, note your efforts to obtain the records, the dates of those efforts, and any administration support in getting records. Start a new cumulative, permanent health card.
- Include all information provided to you in the folder.
- Obtain written permission from the parent(s) to share confidential health information with teachers and other personnel whom you deem appropriate.
- Regardless of whether documentation is done electronically or in hardcopy form, make sure the information is kept secure. Folders should be stored in a locked file cabinet, and your password for electronic data should not be shared. Forward information to a sending school only when written parental permission has been obtained and it is permitted by your district policy. Always use discretion.
- When a student transfers out of your district, keep a copy of the permanent health record for your files.
- Maintain student records for the time designated by your district, usually until the student is 21 years old.
- Alphabetically arrange all files according to class or grade level.
- Keep copies of permanent health forms for all students placed out of the district.
- In some districts all school documents are now computerized. The same rules for privacy apply.

FAST FACTS in a NUTSHELL

Assembling, reviewing, and entering all this information into a permanent record can be very time consuming. When a district does not allocate money for summer work, the task is especially frustrating. You will want to have as much done as possible before students enter yet resent spending your personal time.

Clinical Snapshot

School nurse Adrianna completes as much of her charting as possible before the school year ends. As documents arrive, she starts the students' folders and continuously updates. This way, as much as possible is done in advance.

DAILY LOGS

In addition to the cumulative health record, the school nurse must document all student visits to the health office. Ideally, entries should be made immediately. However, the health office is a busy place, and this is often not possible. The following procedure may help you keep track of numerous visits.

Role of School Nurses in Maintaining Daily Logs

- Use a notebook or clipboard on which students write their names and times of arrival. Young children should bring passes from their teachers that include the date, time, child's name, and teacher observations. These notes are available for all to see, so they should contain no further information. Keep these notes and log pages for each student until he or she has graduated or reaches 21 years of age so you can reference them if necessary in a legal action.
- Assess each student using the nursing process: check vital signs, note skin color and body language, and so on.
- Take a history. Ask relevant questions: *Were you sick this morning? What were you doing in class before coming to my office?*
- Speak with a parent or teacher if necessary.
- At this point, do one of three things:
  - Allow the student to rest and continue to observe him or her.
  - Send the student back to class.
  - Excuse the student from school.
- Check on the student's status later in the day.
- Document your actions on the student's individual log sheet or software standardized form. Include *all* relevant data, conversations, follow-up efforts, and outcome.
- If the incident or illness warrants further clarification, complete an incident report and file it according to district policy.
- Protect all students' privacy. Do not make their complaints known to others in your office. Keep records in their folders and the folders in the locked file cabinet or under your password in whatever software program you are using.

EMERGENCY HEALTH CARDS

Every student and teacher must have an annually updated emergency card. Keep emergency cards in an accessible but secure location. Save the previous year's cards to verify information.

Information Needed on an Emergency Health Card

- Student's name, address, and home phone number
- Parents' names and addresses if different from the student's
- Parents' e-mail addresses, work and cell phone numbers
- Several reliable contact people whom you can call if parents are unavailable
- One parent's or guardian's signature
- Name of the legal custodian(s)
- Physician's name and phone number

The emergency health card can also be used to update health information. Add the following question:

Is there any new information regarding your child's health status? No___ Yes___ Comment:_____.

You may also ask parents to initial a box if they *do not* wish to have health information shared with relevant staff members. This gives you the needed consent in writing.

Include a reminder about the school's medication policy. Add district requirements for returning to school after an illness and the school exclusion policy.

When dealing with an ill child who must be excluded, keep in mind the following:

- Do not allow anyone who is not named on the card to pick up a student unless the parent gives explicit permission. The student should be able to identify that person and appear comfortable with him or her.
- Do not permit a student to leave with anyone he or she does not recognize or whose behavior is inappropriate.
- Always call a parent first regarding illnesses and accidents.
- Do not discuss a student's health problem with anyone who answers the phone at the parent's home or work number.

Role of School Nurses in Keeping Emergency Health Cards

- Be certain that every child and staff member has an annually updated card.
- Make sure cards are all completed accurately and signed by parents or guardians.
- Include a card in the admission packet for newly enrolled students.
- Store cards in a secure area.

===============*FAST FACTS in a NUTSHELL*

Coordinate with nursing colleagues on the keeping and filing of reports. Explore new technology to simplify recordkeeping.

Clinical Snapshot

Adriana is one of several nurses in the district. She needs to collaborate with her district colleagues to unify the approach to paperwork. It will be easier for any substitutes and save time and money in the long run.

ADMINISTRATIVE REPORTS

The school nurse is responsible for a number of reports throughout the school year. Not all reports are required by every school, district, or state. Check with your administration to see what is relevant for you and the date on which any reports are due. Some of the more commonly requested reports are described in the following sections.

Daily, Weekly, Monthly, and Annual Reports

These reports are made upon a request and help justify how you are spending your time. Prepare a checklist of the number of health office visits, exclusions, medications given, phone conferences, screenings performed, deficiency notices sent out, classes taught, and so on. This is an excellent way to communicate with your administrator and keep a record of statistics.

Child Study Team

Every child who is evaluated by the Child Study Team should have input from the school nurse. Prepare a report that includes a summary of the last physical examination and any health problem that could interfere with learning. Attend the meeting to discuss the report, especially if there are significant medical issues.

504 Accommodations

Students with 504 Accommodation Plans have difficulty with one or more activities of daily life. There are children who require accommodations during the school day so that maximum learning can take place. Be aware of these children, know the extent of the required accommodations, and ensure that the accommodations are implemented.

Tuberculosis Report

Most states require some type of report so they can follow up on the incidence of tuberculosis. This is how they evaluate the need for testing in particular areas. Standardized forms asking for the number of students and staff tested, and the results, are usually sent by the state and must be completed by the school nurse.

Immunization Status Report

Once you have completed checking all your students' immunizations, you must file an annual report with the state. It includes information on the number of students with provisional admission as well as those with medical and religious exemptions.

Nursing Service Plan

Some states require an annual quality assurance report. Part of this report asks school nurses to identify those students needing specialized nursing care. It is designed to make sure students with medical needs are cared for adequately.

Role of School Nurses in Filing Administrative Reports

- Know what—and when—reports are due for your district.
- Keep careful records so retrieving the information will be easy.
- Use this information to support your need for more nursing assistance.

ACCIDENT OR INCIDENT REPORTS

An accident or incident report is a written statement by an eyewitness, which is obtained and provided as part of the legal record as close to the time of the event as possible. It is part of the overall risk management program of any institution's policy, including school district policy. Accident or incident reports are generally used postincident to review and evaluate nursing care; to monitor equipment, the grounds, and buildings for unsafe conditions; and to document events in anticipation of insurance claims (Schwab & Gelfman, 2001).

The person who actually witnesses an incident should provide the firsthand information. If no adult observed an incident firsthand, the nurse should document in the form, for example, "Mrs. Smith stated that Robert fell, hitting his head."

Role of School Nurses in Reporting Accidents or Incidents

- Keep in mind the importance of prevention. The school nurse's first task is to anticipate accidents as much as possible. Be involved in risk management and assessment in the building and on the playground.
- Keep the administration informed of potential problems, as well as immediately following an incident.
- Periodically call the local police department to see if injuries have occurred after hours on playground equipment or the

school grounds. If repeated accidents occur on the same equipment it should be evaluated for defects.

- Keep detailed records and reports of all potentially libelous incidents. Any situation that is out of the ordinary should be noted.
- Include only factual information relevant to an incident.
- In addition to an accident report, you must still enter the information on the student's personal log sheet as you would for any health office visit.

8

Children With Special Needs

An anecdote from New England goes like this:

> *A group of children is waiting to enter school early one morning. A surprise snowstorm has made the front steps impassable, and the janitor is shoveling the stairs as the children wait.*
>
> *A small boy in a wheelchair says, "Sir, could you please shovel the ramp so I can get in?"*
>
> *Impatiently, the janitor responds, "These kids are waiting to use the stairs. As soon as I get the steps cleared, I will shovel the ramp. You will have to wait."*
>
> *"But," says the little boy, "if you shovel off the ramp, we can all get in." (Lavoie, 2005)*
>
> *Children with special needs are now, and forever will be, in the building. Federal laws have made this a reality, and it is the job of school nurses to help them succeed. To do this, we must look closely at who these children with special needs are.*

In this chapter, you will learn:

1. Definitions of *impairment, disability, handicap,* and *special needs,* and the history of special education in our country
2. The general provisions of, and major differences between, the Americans with Disabilities Act and the Individuals with Disabilities Education Act, and how they affect children with special needs
3. How to write appropriate Individualized Healthcare and Emergency Health Plans

4. How demonstrating knowledge and compassion for children with special needs and their parents is part of the school nurse's role as health counselor

CHILDREN WITH SPECIAL NEEDS

When we hear that a child has "special needs," we might immediately assume that the child has a physical handicap and is confined to a wheelchair. A wheelchair is a visible sign that accommodations must be made for the child. We step aside, hold open the door, and stand ready to assist in any way possible. The sad truth is that most children with special needs have problems that cannot be seen. A disability may not be readily apparent to casual observers. These children look the same as other children; therefore, they are expected to behave the same.

Impairment

An impairment is some type of problem with body function or structure. An impairment can be physical, sensory, or developmental in nature.

Disability

A disability is the result of an impairment. A physical impairment would be cerebral palsy. Visual or auditory deficits would be considered sensory impairments. Pervasive developmental disorder is developmental in nature. Disability is thus a complex phenomenon in which impairments interfere with the interaction between features of a person's body and features of the societal norms in which he or she lives (World Health Organization, "Disabilities," n.d.). The disability can be:

- Inherited: genetically transmitted
- Congenital: obtained during gestation
- Acquired: through illness or injury
- Of unknown origin

Whether the disability is permanent or transient, mild or severe, in one or multiple areas, the student will have difficulty behaving and learning in the same way as his or her peers.

Handicap

A child with a handicap has a disadvantage in some way that makes achievement unusually difficult. Academic success can be impeded by hearing or vision loss. A child who is emotionally disturbed will not be able to function to his or her full capacity.

Special Needs

This is an umbrella term that includes children with medical, behavioral, developmental, learning, or mental health issues. These issues cover a wide array of diagnoses.

FAST FACTS in a NUTSHELL

Recent years have brought tremendous progress in diagnosing and educating the student with special needs of a physical nature, but we still may not recognize the full potential of the child with mental disabilities.

Clinical Snapshot

Two students in the third grade have special needs. Maria has cerebral palsy and walks with a typical scissor gait. Michael has Asperger's syndrome and is socially compromised. School nurse Emily notices that classmates are overly indulgent in helping Maria navigate about the room but completely intolerant of Michael's behavior. Emily realizes that this is an ideal time and age to speak with and demonstrate acceptance of those with mental special needs. She works with the classroom teacher to educate children in how they can approach, befriend, and accept Michael as a unique member of their class.

The specifics of what caused the special need are well beyond the scope of this book, and, in reality, are of little relevance. A person's brain might be wired differently, his or her body may not perform competently, and he or she may or may not look different from others. Regardless of the problem, it cannot be changed. The condition exists, and a child's disability may have an impact on his or her school performance. The school nurse is part of the team whose task is to maximize these students' educational experience, help them avoid complications, and ideally, enable the student to blend into the school community. Accomplishing this is a significant challenge.

Delegation of Tasks

Today's advances in health care and current legislation have enabled children with increasingly complex behavioral and medical needs to be part of the mainstream. It may be necessary for the school nurse to delegate some of the responsibility for their care.

The American Nurses Association has defined nursing delegation as the transferring of responsibility for performing a nursing activity to another person while retaining accountability for the outcome (ANA & the National Council of State Boards of Nursing, 2013).

Delegation should occur on a case-by-case basis within the parameters of the state laws that regulate nursing practice.

Delegation to unlicensed assistive personnel should be considered when a child's medical condition warrants immediate attention, as with anaphylaxis. The school nurse provides the necessary training and supervision. Today most states permit school nurses to train delegates for epinephrine and glucagon administration.

Healthy People 2020 Objectives

Disability and Health, 14

Increase the proportion of children and youth with disabilities who spend at least 80% of their time in regular educational programs from 56.8% in 2007–2008 to 73.8%.

HISTORY OF SPECIAL EDUCATION

The history of how society has treated those with special needs is *not* one to be proud of. In the early 1800s, many people were superstitious about those who had mental or physical disabilities. Parents who had the emotional and financial resources kept such children at home and simply managed as best they could. Ashamed of their offspring, parents without resources sometimes abandoned these children and allowed them to die, believing that these "bad" children might be possessed by the devil.

The later 1800s saw the beginnings of institutions for persons with special needs. The objectives were clear. These people were to be given humane treatment, yet kept apart from "normal" people. Education was not even a consideration.

Once compulsory school attendance was mandated in the early 1900s, states were forced to recognize the large numbers of students with special needs. Such children could still be excluded, but by gathering together, these children and their parents began to have a voice. That voice grew stronger and soon demanded to be heard by lawmakers.

According to data from the National Center for Educational Statistics, in 2011 to 2012, 6.4 million students, or 13% of the student population, were receiving special education. (National Center for Educational Statistics, 2014). Many more children were not receiving special education services but needed some type of classroom accommodations.

FAST FACTS in a NUTSHELL

If you have a self-contained special education class in your building, try to spend time in it. Ask to be included in some of their activities so the children will be comfortable with you.

Clincal Snapshot

School nurse Emily suggests that when children are ready to be mainstreamed they start in her health class. Emily is aware of each child's special needs and is able to deal with them appropriately. Depending on the area of need and the class, small group activities can be arranged to provide acceptance and learning opportunities for all.

LEGISLATION

In the early 1970s, public consciousness of people with disabilities was raised. Before that time, there were few educational choices for children with special needs. By 1975, two pieces of federal legislation were in place that had a significant impact on the educational process of special needs students:

- Section 504 of the Rehabilitation Act
- The Education for All Handicapped Children Act

In 1990, those laws were amended and expanded to include even more services for children with special needs. Today, they are known as the Americans with Disabilities Act (ADA), P.L. 101–336, and the Individuals with Disabilities Education Act (IDEA), P.L. 101–476.

Both laws broaden and define the services offered to children with special needs. Table 8.1 provides a historical perspective on the laws that have affected students with special needs.

Provisions of the Americans With Disabilities Act and Section 504 Services

Americans with Disabilities Act

The ADA is a broad civil rights law. It protects the rights of all persons with disabilities. Students are eligible if they have a physical or mental impairment that limits one or more major life activities: learning, breathing, walking, eating, and so on. A multidisciplinary accommodation team must be available to determine eligibility. The team then formulates a plan that describes the nature of the disability and how the student is to be accommodated. For instance, accommodations might include hearing devices or medication for allergic reactions or asthma.

TABLE 8.1 Timeline of Major Legislation Affecting Students With Special Needs

1791	Tenth Amendment of the U.S. Constitution gives individual states authority in educational matters.
1880	National Education Association and Office of Education are created and initiate an age–grade-level system categorizing students according to age. Differences in children become apparent quickly.
1919	All states require compulsory school attendance.
1954	U.S. Supreme Court rules on *Brown vs. Board of Education,* putting an end to "separate but equal" schools. The rights of individual diversity are emphasized and will serve to influence future rulings regarding children with special needs in school.
1961	Special Education Act, P.L. 87–276, authorizes federal money to train teachers of children who are deaf.
1965	Elementary and Secondary Education Act, P.L. 89–10, is the first in a sequence of federal laws to require educational opportunities for students with handicapping conditions.

(continued)

	TABLE 8.1 Timeline of Major Legislation Affecting Students With Special Needs (*continued*)
1973	Section 504 of the Rehabilitation Act, P.L. 93–112, bars discrimination against people with disabilities in any federally funded program and requires appropriate education services for children who are disabled. It mandates access to all public buildings for anyone with a disability.
1975	Education for All Handicapped Children Act, P.L. 94–142, mandates a free and appropriate public education for all children with disabilities. This is the core of funding for special education. It requires that accommodations be made in the public school setting to ensure that educational opportunities are the same for all.
1990	Americans with Disabilities Act, P.L. 101–336, based on the Rehabilitation Act of 1973, is passed and guarantees equal opportunities for persons with disabilities. Physical barriers must be removed and all new construction must be made accessible to those with disabilities.
1990	Individuals with Disabilities Education Act, P.L. 101–476, formerly the Education for All Handicapped Children Act, expands services and adds additional categories of children eligible to receive services.

Individualized Healthcare Plan

It is up to the school nurse to determine whether a child is in need of an Individualized Healthcare Plan (IHP). Unlike an Individualized Education Plan (IEP), which is mandated by law and educationally based, an IHP is developed solely to provide the nurse a way to recognize health care needs, document the provision of care, and progress toward achieving desired outcomes. It simplifies communication with other professionals.

504 Accommodation Plan

Students not meeting the criteria for IDEA services can be considered for services under Section 504 of the Rehabilitation Act of 1973. To be eligible the student must have a physical or mental impairment that substantially limits one or more major life activities—breathing, walking, eating, and so on.

It is your responsibility to write and update the Emergency Care Plan and Individualized Healthcare Plan annually. Books available through your state and national association provide samples you can modify to meet each student's unique needs.

🌀 Clincal Snapshot

Jon is a 6-year-old severely diabetic student. His blood sugar levels are unstable and he needs frequent testing. Emily has developed an IHP that includes an accurate assessment, nursing diagnosis, anticipated outcomes, nursing interventions, and means to evaluate. Emily then formulates an ECP with specific directions indicating what to do in the event of a school emergency.

If Jon's classification is included in any of the categories under IDEA below, the 504 Accommodation Plan or IHP can be part of the IEP.

Emergency Care Plan

If necessary, an ECP should also be developed to address specific actions to be taken for a child who has a classroom emergency. This plan includes parent and physician contact information and states simply, "If this happens, do this."

Provisions of the Individuals with Disabilities Education Act (IDEA)

IDEA provides funding for children with educationally handicapping conditions. Students who fit into one of the categories of disabilities identified below are eligible for services:

Autism	Orthopedic impairment
Deaf-blindness	Other health impairment
Deafness	Specific learning disability
Emotional disturbance	Speech/language impairment
Hearing impairment	Traumatic brain injury
Intellectual disability	Visual impairment
Multiple disabilities	

IDEA reinforces provisions adapted from the Education for All Handicapped Children Act. It includes the following components:

- *A free and appropriate public education for all:* All services must be provided without cost to parents or guardians.
- *The right of due process:* Parents have legal recourse if they are dissatisfied with their children's education.
- *Education in the least restrictive environment:* Mainstreaming, inclusion, and pull-out practices are used to keep the students with special needs in the classroom with peers as much as possible.
- *IEP:* Each child has a specific plan appropriate for his or her needs.

An IEP is written and designed specifically for students with special needs by the Child Study Team. It includes goals and short-term objectives stated in instructional terms. It must include support services to be provided and justification for any special placement recommended. It must be periodically evaluated.

IDEA expanded support services to include transportation; early detection initiatives; related physical, occupational, and speech therapies; and assistive technology devices.

To meet these criteria, districts are required to have a Child Study Team composed of the classroom teacher; the special education teacher; an administrator; a parent or guardian; a learning disability specialist; a psychologist; a social worker; a physical, speech, or occupational therapist; and the school nurse.

Differences Between IDEA and Section 504

IDEA requires each state to set up a process to address the law. Section 504 is a civil rights law that prohibits discrimination based on handicaps. Federal funds are provided for children classified under IDEA, whereas no federal funds are provided for 504 accommodations. School districts must bear costs for 504 accommodations. All students who are considered to be disabled under IDEA need some type of accommodation to succeed. They must fit into one of the categories to be eligible for services. These same children will need accommodations that will be covered in their IEPs. IDEA addresses only those with specific conditions. Section 504 addresses all children with handicaps in activities of daily living.

Areas of Comparison	IDEA	Section 504
Federal law	Yes	Yes
Due process	Set up by state	Governed by federal law
Funding	Federal funding	No federal funding; school district bears the cost
Accommodation required	All eligible students must fit into a specific category of disability (IEP); those eligible must be accommodated for specific conditions	All students who are unable to perform one or more activities of daily life must be accommodated

Levels of Acuity (Washington State Model)

Children with special needs may require a greater amount of, and more, specialized nursing care in the school setting than do other children. These children are usually classified under IDEA or have a 504 Accommodation Plan. They are placed in one of four categories:

Level I	Nursing dependent	Requires nursing care 24 hours a day (e.g., ventilator dependent)
Level II	Medically fragile	Has possibility of life-threatening emergency (e.g., severely diabetic, seizure disorder)
Level III	Medically complex	Requires daily treatment or close monitoring (e.g., asthma, attention deficit hyperactivity disorder)
Level IV	Health concerns	Occasional monitoring (e.g., migraines, eating disorders)

Some possible reasons for an increase in the number of children identified as having special needs include the following:

• Improved methods of detection
• Better survival rates for infants at risk
• Increased survival of infants from low-weight multiple births with early developmental issues
• The broadening of diagnostic categories encompassing more children

THE SCHOOL NURSE AS A HEALTH COUNSELOR

Working with children with special needs and their parents is probably the greatest challenge faced by school nurses. We have been well trained and can easily tend to their physical needs: catheterizations, tube feedings, medications, nebulizer treatments, and so on. It is the emotional care that is absolutely draining.

The parents may be angry. They might mourn their child's lost potential and their own unfulfilled dreams. Parents are not always happy about what school personnel have to say and may choose to vent their wrath on the school, and the school nurse in particular. Much of special education is funded by the federal government, but some is not. Even one child can financially burden a district and financially ruin a family. Often, parents have to fight for services, and lawsuits can be involved, creating justifiable tension.

FAST FACTS in a NUTSHELL

There is no single correct way of providing care for children with special needs. The school nurse must remain an objective, nonjudgmental, and up-to-date resource and remember that the best decision is always the one that will provide the best benefit to the child. Be mindful that no one, not even you, will be able to fix the source of the problem.

Clinical Snapshot

School nurse Emily is caught between the parents' wishes and district recommendations for placement of a special needs child. Out-of-district placement, busing, and private placement are extremely expensive for any school district. The district is adamant that the child's needs can be met within district. Emily feels strongly that the child's medical issues are so overwhelming they would best be addressed in an out-of-district placement. Emily makes her feelings known, in writing, to the Child Study Team and works to find a comfortable compromise.

ROLE OF SCHOOL NURSES RELATED TO CHILDREN WITH SPECIAL NEEDS

- Know and understand the laws relevant to special education.
- Establish a comfortable, supportive relationship with parents.
- Identify children with special needs as early as possible.
- Help children with special needs blend into the school community.
- Advocate for these children.
- Develop health-related IEP goals.
- Secure signed, written releases for confidential information.
- Develop and implement 504 Accommodation Plans, IHPs, and ECPs.
- Serve as a liaison among students, teachers, parents, and health care providers.
- Identify and utilize community resources.
- Delegate, train, and supervise paraprofessional staff in the delivery of special nursing procedures according to state and school district policies.
- Get out of your centrally located, well-ventilated office and . . . *"Shovel the ramp!"*

9

School Law

The surest way to get hired for a school nurse position is to stress the fact that you will carefully follow school policies and procedures to keep your district within the law. The surest way not to get hired is to be totally naive about the very real possibility that you could be involved in a lawsuit. Unfortunately, schools are always under scrutiny and the school nurse is frequently at the forefront of a pending lawsuit.

Today's school is a complex legal environment. You will learn quickly that nothing is more important to a board of education than feeling totally comfortable knowing that the school nurse is aware of the basic legal framework governing schools and will be protectively proactive for the district and himself or herself.

In this chapter, you will learn:

1. The three levels of laws
2. Elements of the different classifications of laws
3. Distinctions among liability, negligence, and malpractice
4. Major areas of potential liability and strategies to avoid lawsuits

LEVELS OF LAWS

Laws are written and enacted at three levels: federal, state, and local.

Federal Laws

In 1791, the Tenth Amendment of the U.S. Constitution gave authority to the individual states in educational matters. Federal laws and policies usually defer to state and local governments, provided that they do not violate any constitutional rights.

The federal government collaborates with state and local school districts to improve public education. The federal government may fund educational programs contingent on the implementation of specific policies.

State Laws

The state has the authority to act in the interest of protecting the citizens of that state. The state has significant power to determine minimum attendance requirements, curricula, and educational requirements. Since passage of the Tenth Amendment in 1791, states have had full and complete jurisdiction in educational matters and can delegate certain power to local school districts.

Local Laws

All states have district school boards of education whose members are either appointed by local government officials or elected by popular vote. These boards of education can determine the specific content of curricula, raise funds, and hire personnel. The local district determines the instructional methods and materials to be used to best meet their students' needs.

CLASSIFICATIONS OF LAWS

There are three basic classifications of laws in the United States: criminal, civil, and administrative. School nurses need to know the parameters of each classification.

Criminal Laws

These are statutes enacted to maintain order and protect society as a whole. There are, for example, laws against the crimes of theft, illegal drug use, libel, slander, medical malpractice, practicing without a license, failing to report child abuse, tampering with official records, and kidnapping.

Civil Laws

These laws protect the rights of the individual. Enforcement of civil laws often involves an attempt to find a peaceable resolution through compensation or by stopping the actionable practice. The Family Educational Rights and Privacy Act (FERPA) of 1974 and the Health Insurance Portability and Accountability Act (HIPAA) of 1996 are examples of civil laws.

Family Educational Rights and Privacy Act

FERPA is a federal law that protects the privacy of student educational records. It applies to all schools that receive funds under an applicable program of the U.S. Department of Education. The act contains the following provisions:

- Parents have the right to access their children's educational records.
- All school records are considered educational.
- Personally identifiable student information contained in health records must be protected.
- Sensitive records, such as those concerning child abuse, and psychological and counseling information, should be kept separate and secure.
- Access is limited to those with a "legitimate educational interest."
- Student files kept on computers must have safeguards in place to ensure the same level of security.
- Parental consent is required before records can be transferred to a new school.

Health Insurance Portability and Accountability Act

HIPAA was written to address the concern of maintaining the confidentiality of health records transmitted electronically. Among its key provisions are the following:

- The primary goal is to make it easier for people to retain health insurance, protect confidentiality, and help control administrative costs in health care.
- There are two separate sections: Title I deals with portability, allowing individuals to carry health insurance from one job to another. Title II deals with administrative simplification by

setting standards for receiving, transmitting, and maintaining health care information and ensuring privacy.

- Compliance is focused on health care providers or agencies that bill the individual.
- HIPAA provides that patients have a right to receive notice of the privacy practices of the provider.
- It was not intended to interfere with the sharing of necessary health information between the school and health care providers. Schools and physicians are considered "covered entities," and information can be shared on a "need-to-know" basis. Written permission from the parent is required.

Administrative Laws

Criminal and civil laws determine what can or cannot be done in particular situations.

Administrative laws determine who will interpret, enforce, and regulate laws. Agencies such as state boards of nursing are given the responsibility of handling such statutory laws pertaining to nursing. They have the authority to revoke nurses' licenses when nurses have not met the standards of care set forth by the state's nurse practice act (Selekman, 2006, p. 298).

LIABILITY, NEGLIGENCE, AND MALPRACTICE

To be *liable* for something is to be responsible for one's own conduct. In our schools today, two principles should guide our actions: *reasonableness* and *in loco parentis*. Nurses and teachers are expected to act in a *reasonable* fashion. *In loco parentis* means "in place of the parent." This identifies the protective relationship of nurses and teachers to students. It justifies their ability and responsibility to take care of students' needs.

A nurse is considered *negligent* if he or she fails to act in a manner in which another nurse in a similar situation would have acted, and his or her performance falls below a reasonable *standard of care*. For the school nurse, the degree of care that another prudent school nurse under the same set of circumstances would have rendered indicates whether an action was negligent.

Malpractice is negligence by a professional person, such as a physician or nurse.

School districts carry the necessary malpractice insurance to cover employees. School nurses are included in this coverage. However, many nurses carry their own individual malpractice insurance because of the additional benefits provided, which cover them whether or not they are working in the school.

Clinical Snapshot

School nurse Beverly has been employed by the same district for more than 10 years. She also works per diem at the local community hospital. Both school and hospital cover her while she is employed; however, Beverly, also carries a separate policy that covers her individually for all other nursing services and provides added protection should she be sued in any capacity.

LEGAL ISSUES AND THE COORDINATED SCHOOL HEALTH PROGRAM

As mentioned in Chapter 1, the coordinated school health program includes eight components that cover all areas of student and staff needs. These areas are used as a reference point by Collins, Goodman, and Moulton (2008) in their Centers for Disease Control and Prevention review of what the laws require of schools. A summary of some potential liability issues are identified for each component, along with suggested strategies that school nurses can use to avoid legal encounters.

Health Education

- *Issues:* Health lessons on sensitive topics such as sexuality, emotional health, and substance abuse.
- *Strategies:* Work within your approved health curriculum. Never ask personal questions. Make sure you receive proper training. Send home written notices of topics to be covered. Allow parents the opportunity to review the curriculum and exclude their child.

Physical Education and Activity

Issues: Equal opportunity to participate in sports for both sexes, adaptive physical education, Individualized Education Plans (IEPs) and Individualized Healthcare Plans (IHPs), sports injuries, protective gear, proper supervision, staff training in cardiopulmonary resuscitation (CPR) and use of *automated external defibrillators* (AED), and gym participation exemptions

Strategies: Check that sport activities are offered for girls. Review IEPs and IHPs to make sure students with special needs receive adaptive physical education if included in their IEP. See that helmets, safety glasses, and so on are available and worn. Look into the student–teacher ratio of physical education classes. Offer CPR/AED classes to physical education teachers and any other staff member who requests certification.

Exemptions and restrictions must be clarified by a physician and honored by physical education teachers. Check dates and types of restrictions. Use caution in allowing students to return to full activity. Keep physical education teachers informed of students with restrictions and of when they are cleared to return to class.

FAST FACTS in a NUTSHELL

Even if a student has been cleared for return to full participation in physical education, consider the anticipated activity.

Clinical Snapshot

Lisa, age 6, was casted for 6 weeks following a fracture in her right wrist. She presents a note from her orthopedist stating that she is cleared to return to gym and allowed to participate in all activities. School nurse Beverly is aware that Lisa's physical education class will be doing exercises using the monkey bars. She can suggest that Lisa avoid this specific activity for a few more weeks knowing it will place tremendous strain on her newly healed wrist.

Health Services

- *Issues:* First aid, emergency care, medications, screenings, routine and sports assessments, privacy, child abuse, communicable diseases, and students with special needs

- *Strategies:* Have annually updated, signed standing orders, IEPs, and Emergency Care Plans. Maintain current CPR/AED certifications. Carefully note health issues, especially heart defects, chronic conditions, seizure disorders, and so on. Include actions to be taken for a classroom emergency. Perform and accurately document first aid and medication administration according to school policy and procedures. Administer only medications that must be given in school. Attend and be vocal at Child Study Team meetings. Follow up on all screening referrals. Report suspicion of child abuse to the proper agency. Know and report rare infectious diseases as required by local policy. Report high levels of communicable diseases to county and state authorities.

FAST FACTS in a NUTSHELL

If a child has a known cardiac condition for which he or she is being followed by a cardiologist, request that the cardiologist, not the pediatrician, clear him or her for participation in physical education.

Clinical Snapshot

School nurse Beverly enrolls a new student from an Asian country. The physical examination form has been signed by a local pediatrician and returned, indicating that the student is cleared for all activity. However, in reviewing a previous physical exam record from the student's country of origin, Beverly sees a notation indicating that he had a period of apnea at 18 months. Beverly knows that the pediatrician is not fluent in the student's first language and questions whether this information was shared during the most recent examination. Beverly suggests an interpreter return with the parents and sends a copy of the previous physical examination. If Beverly is not satisfied that the cardiac condition is addressed properly, she can discuss the student with the school physician before permitting the child to participate in physical education.

Nutrition Services

- *Issues:* Anaphylaxis, nutritious lunch offerings, cleanliness and behavior in the lunchroom, and rights of children with food allergies

- *Strategies:* Educate lunchroom staff about signs and symptoms of anaphylaxis. Keep an epinephrine autoinjector available, Check that dietary regulations are followed. Form a committee of parents of children with food allergies. Consider their input on how to protect their children while allowing socialization. Insist on adequate lunchroom supervision. Hang a poster demonstrating the Heimlich maneuver in the lunchroom and annually train the lunchroom aides in how to administer it.

Mental Health and Social Services

- *Issues:* Child neglect and abuse, mental health problems (e.g., depression, suicide)
- *Strategies:* If required, see that counseling services are provided. Know your students and your limitations. Immediately report any suspicions of child abuse, depression, and suicidal thoughts expressed by students. Do not try to treat or counsel these students. Work with other professionals in the district to get the students professional help.

Healthful and Safe School Environment

- *Issues:* Indoor air quality, noise, physical security of the building, heating, air conditioning, asbestos, radon, lead contamination in drinking water, injuries caused by unsafe equipment, fire drills, maintenance of fire extinguishers and detectors, school bus safety, pedestrian safety, violence, locker searches, substance abuse, alcohol use, inappropriate student–staff relationships, and school disasters
- *Strategies:* Refer complaints of environmental issues immediately, and follow up. Question whether proper inspections have been made for drinking fountains, asbestos, playground equipment safety, and so on. Look into school bus safety, seat belt availability, and supervision. Insist on a no-bullying, no-violence policy. Report and document all violent behavior and bullying incidents. Do not become involved in any search of a student for drugs or weapons, whether the student is dressed or undressed.

Health Promotion for Staff

- *Issues:* Physical exams, privacy, 504 accommodations

- *Strategies:* Cooperate with the administration in obtaining physical examinations of employees. Store files in the most secure location. Administer and follow up on tuberculosis testing. Provide recommendations for 504 accommodations for staff as needed. Remain a health resource for staff. Be discreet about staff personal issues.

Parent/Family and Community Involvement

- *Issues:* Policy and decision-making dilemmas, parental consent for certain services, and privacy concerns
- *Strategies:* Encourage partnerships with parent and community groups. Solicit parent involvement as much as possible. Communicate frequently with parents via newsletters, meetings, and office visits. Remain accessible.

FAST FACTS in a NUTSHELL

You may also have legal council provided through your teacher's union. Explore your possible sources before a need arises.

Clincal Snapshot

Beverly is employed as a school nurse under a teacher's contract and has union dues deducted annually from her pay. She checks with her union leader and learns that she is entitled to 30 minutes of legal advice in any area she needs—home purchase, divorce, writing a will, and so on.

ROLE OF SCHOOL NURSES IN SCHOOL LAW

- Know and remain current on the laws relevant to your district, state, and country.
- Seek legal advice as needed.
- Remain flexible so you can adapt to religious and ethnic diversities.
- Document and save all correspondence from parents, colleagues, students, outside agencies, and so on.
- Maintain professionalism.
- Notify appropriate people in writing of legal concerns.
- Practice preventive strategies to avoid legal problems.

10

High-Risk Areas
in School Nursing Practice

Every day, the school nurse must decide how best to handle certain situations. He or she has standing orders for routine care and for Individualized Healthcare and Emergency Care Plans that address students with specific needs. However, for people on the front lines of the health care delivery system, many situations can arise that have no definitive right or wrong resolution. States, school districts, and professional ethics may be in conflict. Families and communities differ, as resources, values, and expectations are unique to every person and vary by community. What is acceptable in one school, community, or state may not be acceptable in another.

In this chapter, you will learn:

1. The reasons school nurses are at a high risk for liability
2. How to balance the responsibilities of the nursing profession and school policies
3. Areas of conflict in school nursing practice

HIGH-RISK ASPECTS OF SCHOOL HEALTH NURSING PRACTICE

Certain aspects of school health practices put school nurses at higher risk for liability than their colleagues in some other settings, including the following:

- Professional isolation
- A wide range of responsibilities
- Conflicts between policies of boards of education and professional standards of care
- Conflicts between education law and health law (Schwab & Gelfman, 2001, p. 77)

FAST FACTS in a NUTSHELL

A school setting is quite different from a hospital. In an acute care setting, a nurse is surrounded by other competent health professionals, has access to diagnostic equipment, and is in an acute care mindset. In contrast, seldom does a school nurse work with another nurse of equal stature, and never is there a physician on site. Available equipment consists of a thermometer, stethoscope, and blood pressure machine. The focus is on prevention rather than intervention.

Clinical Snapshot

School nurse Andrea is summoned from lunch to evaluate a student, Katherine, who is 10 years old. She had gone to the principal's office stating, *I can't breathe*. The principal panicked and immediately called for Andrea. When Andrea arrives, she notes that Katherine's color is fine, her air exchange is good, and respirations are easy at 20. Andrea gives her water and allows her to rest. While talking with Katherine, Andrea learns she has been excluded from a circle of girls and is very unhappy. Andrea summons the other girls to talk about the cruel behavior and privately discuss the overreaction with Katherine.

Consider a child who is truly in respiratory distress and is brought to the emergency room. Some time has already lapsed since the first symptom appeared, and numerous people have already seen the patient. An assessment has been made, and it was determined that immediate care was needed at a hospital facility.

The hospital staff then address these needs and intervene to choose the level of care required. The pulse-oxygen level is checked immediately, and oxygen can be started. An intravenous infusion with appropriate medication or a nebulizer, or both, will be administered. Blood will be drawn and sent out stat. All personnel are prepared to perform cardiopulmonary resuscitation if needed.

In contrast, in the school setting, the nurse must assess alone with limited diagnostic tools. He or she might call for an ambulance without being certain that a student is indeed in distress. Perhaps this is a student who frequently seeks out the school nurse. Did an embarrassing incident trigger a dramatic reaction in the student? Is the distress caused by a reason totally unrelated to illness? Would a drink of water, a puff from an inhaler, or a little downtime and some kind words be all the student needs?

The school nurse has very few minutes to process all of these possibilities. How accurately you make assessments and appropriate decisions, and balance your numerous tasks, will depend largely on the type and years of your nursing experience, educational preparation, and personal, professional, and ethical beliefs.

FAST FACTS in a NUTSHELL

School nurses have already had some hospital or acute-care experience. School experience will come in time, but each situation in the school setting is unique and requires individualized care and attention.

Clinical Snapshot

Mary Beth is one of those students who needs to see you every day. She is a 10th grader with an unstable home life who always appears sad. Today she complains of vague *stomach pains*. School nurse Andrea allows her to stay and tries to engage her in conversation. Her affect is different and you note her poor color. When Andrea palpates her abdomen, she indicates tenderness. Playing it safe, Andrea calls home and suggest she be seen immediately by a physician.

Your educational level will depend on what the law requires in the state in which you practice. However, all professionals must continue to learn. If you do not have the skills required for the school setting, you must get them: from nursing colleagues, an acute care setting, continuing education, or an academic program in a college or university. Each state has its own board of nursing and nurse practice act defining the scope of practice, but some issues vary across state lines.

The school nurse's job is multifaceted and little understood by other school personnel. While you are attempting to assess a child with respiratory symptoms, other children may continue to arrive for their medications, a diabetic student may need to be tested, and no one else will be available to do these tasks. There are always myriad opportunities for errors to be made. In spite of this overwhelming responsibility, there are teachers and administrators who believe that unless you are teaching 25 students all day, every day, you are not working. A great deal of what school nurses do must be held in confidence; consequently, few people truly know (or care) how you fill your days.

The school nurse stands with one foot in each discipline: nursing and education. As nurses, we must abide by our state's nurse practice act, as the state board of nursing issues our licenses. As teachers, we are employed by the local board of education and obliged to heed federal, state, and district regulations regarding educational matters.

In truth, we serve many masters: several layers of government, our nursing profession, school principals, directors of special services, state boards of nursing, teachers' unions, parents, and so on.

NEGLIGENCE

Negligence cases against school nurses are usually based on allegations that an action taken (or not taken) does not meet the current standards of care. This means that another competent nurse would not have acted in the same way. Some examples of negligence include failure to:

- Keep abreast of current nursing knowledge
- Document adequately
- Recognize urgent and emergency situations
- Follow school district policy
- Challenge administrative decisions that put students at risk (Schwab & Gelfman, 2001, p. 77)

The following are theoretical scenarios highlighting some of the dilemmas faced by today's school nurses. As has been mentioned, there are no right or wrong solutions. These scenarios are intended simply to provoke thoughtful discussions.

Issue: Health Office Coverage

Conflict: Nurse practice act versus local board of education

Scenario: A second grader, Emily, is sent to you at 9:55 a.m. and is obviously acutely ill. You are expected to teach a health lesson to her class at 10:00 a.m. You have 5 minutes to assess, call her parent, and get to class.

Discussion Points:

- If you are late to your class, the teacher will not get his or her full preparation time, as granted in his or her (and your) contract. The teacher could file a grievance.
- Was this child sent to school ill, and why did the teacher not send her to you earlier?
- Should you:
  - Bring Emily with you and assess her after class?
  - Take her temperature quickly, call a parent, and have her wait to be picked up in the main office, perhaps excluding a well child or exposing the secretary and others to illness?
  - Stay with her, assess her properly, and allow her to rest on your cot until she feels better and can return to class or until the parent arrives?
  - Make up the health class at a later time in the day or week instead of doing what you had originally planned to do at that time?
  - See if someone else can teach your health class? (Good luck!)

Issue: Clearance to Participate in Sports

Conflict: Private physician versus school physician

Scenario: You note on Luke's assessment record that he has a history of a mild concussion at age 10. He is now a high school senior and you know that he has had at least two other head injuries during soccer games. His private physician has cleared him to participate in football. You report this to the school physician, who refuses to allow him to participate in football. The principal and Luke's parents are angry with you for "making such a big deal" about his history of head injuries.

Discussion Points:

- Who has ultimate authority in decisions like this?
- Should you have raised the question?
- Is there a school policy to back up the exclusion?
- Is the coach given input?
- Can you legally refuse to sign clearance, along with the school physician?
- How will your decision affect your tenure and your job?
- Are you willing to risk the unrest your decision will cause?

Issue: Child Abuse

Conflict: Ethical beliefs versus local district policy

Scenario: Maria is a 12-year-old special education student who, following a class on puberty, tearfully confides to you that her 19-year-old mentally challenged cousin fondles her when they are alone. Maria likes her cousin and denies having had intercourse or ever being forced to allow him to touch her. She begs you to keep this in confidence and swears she will never be alone with her cousin again. Maria fears that her father will physically harm both her cousin and her if he finds out.

Discussion Points:

- Who should address this situation: the school guidance counselor or administration, the children's protective services agency, or the parents?
- Will outside agency involvement cause upheaval in their close Hispanic family?
- As both parties are special education students involved in consensual acts, is this a reportable issue?
- Should you agree to keep Maria's confidence and privately work with the parents?
- How much involvement is it appropriate for you to have?

Issue: Immunizations

Conflict: National and state laws versus state health department and local district policy

Scenario: A family has just immigrated to the United States from a war-torn country. They arrive at the school to register their children but have no health records or immunization documentation. You are fairly certain that they are illegal residents.

Discussion Points:

- As all students are entitled to a free and public education, should you find a clinic to provide immunizations and other health services for the family?
- The family does not have a record of any vaccines. Should you exclude them until they can provide evidence of beginning a series of vaccinations?
- Should you stall as long as possible, as you believe that they will probably move anyway?
- Can you share your suspicions of the family's nonresidency status with the administration?

Issue: Do-Not-Resuscitate Order

Conflict: Personal and professional ethics versus parental orders

Scenario: Catherine is a seventh grader in the final stages of cancer. Her parents have refused further treatment and have requested that no heroic measures be offered. Catherine is to attend school as long as possible, and her parents willingly signed a do-not-resuscitate order.

Discussion Points:

- Can you watch a child stop breathing and stand by without attempting to help her?
- Are these parents setting the school up for legal action?
- If you do nothing, will this result in a lawsuit anyway?
- Are the parents justified in refusing further treatment?
- How can you protect this child while she is in school?
- How can you help the teachers and classmates deal with this tragic situation?

Issue: Confidentiality

Conflict: Teachers' need to know versus parental rights

Scenario: Eduardo is 11 years old and has a seizure disorder that is well controlled with medication that you administer daily at noon. His parents refuse to sign permission for you to share this information with his teachers or anyone else.

Discussion Points:

- How will you prepare Eduardo's teachers for a possible emergency without telling them about his history of seizures?
- Where and how will you document his diagnosis and medication use?
- How will you balance the teachers' need to know with the parents' right to privacy?
- Should you share this information with the school physician and the administration?

Issue: Emergency Treatment

Conflict: Nurse practice act versus local district policy

Scenario: Jacob is brought to your office by the physical education teacher with an audible wheeze and diaphoresis and is clearly struggling to breathe. He has no history of airway obstructive disease. You direct the teacher to call for an ambulance and listen to Jacob's lungs. You clearly hear very poor air exchange and recognize his immediate need for a bronchodilator. You have on hand a nebulizer, tubing, mask, and another student's medication. The paramedics are at least 10 minutes away, and your standing orders do not cover you to medicate in this instance.

Discussion Points:

- Should you try to calm Jacob down, give him water and wait, hoping that his symptoms lessen?
- Are you comfortable enough with your assessment skills to go ahead with the treatment?
- Are you subjecting yourself to a possible lawsuit either way?
- Should you try to call Jacob's physician, and lose valuable time, to get verbal permission to treat him?

Healthy People 2020 Objectives

Respiratory Diseases, 3.1

Reduce the emergency department visits for asthma among children and adults aged 5 to 64 years from 57.0% per 10,000 in 2005–2007 to 49.7% per 10,000

Issue: Administrator Responsibility

Conflict: Administrative authority versus nurse practice act

Scenario: Kevin falls from the top of the monkey bars and hits his head during the lunchtime recess. He is brought to your office complaining of a headache and appears to be stunned. You notice that his pupils are not equally reactive to light. You begin to call for an ambulance. The principal admonishes you, telling you that you are overreacting and should call a parent first to carry out his or her wishes.

Discussion Points:

- Should you listen to the principal?
- Should you call a parent and discuss the situation further with the principal?
- Do you have any written procedure for head injuries?

Issue: Searches

Conflict: Privacy rights versus local school district policy

Scenario: You arrive at your high school one morning and are told that you are to assist with a locker search for drugs and weapons. You ask if there is cause for concern and are not given any information.

Discussion Points:

- As the school nurse, should you be part of this process?
- Have students and parents been informed of the search?
- Should you help without additional information?
- If requested, should you search students' bodies for drugs or weapons?

ROLE OF SCHOOL NURSES IN HIGH-RISK AREAS

- Recognize high-risk areas.
- Be proactive and anticipate dilemmas.
- Seek additional educational preparation as needed. If you have not had acute care experience, get it.
- Stay connected to nursing colleagues and professional organizations.
- Keep careful records; document accurately and appropriately.
- Stay in acute care mode. Be alert for any emergency.

FAST FACTS in a NUTSHELL

The school nurse must deal alone with many controversial areas. Seek to gain trust and confidence from parents, administration, and the school board so that they will support your efforts in any situation, regardless of outcome.

Clinical Snapshot

School nurse Andrea has no standing orders to give acetaminophen or ibuprofen. A 16-year-old female student arrives in her office complaining of dizziness. The student's oral temperature is 103.8°F. Andrea immediately has her lie down; puts cold compresses on her head, axilla, and groin; removes her sneakers; gives a large glass of water; and administers an appropriate dose of liquid ibuprofen. Within a few minutes, the temperature is down and the student feels better. Andrea calls the student's mom and confesses giving medication without permission. She also informs the principal and school doctor. All are grateful, and Andrea subsequently has ibuprofen added to the list of medications she may give for a temperature above 102°F.

- Remember that the school administrator is not licensed to assess a child, you are.
- Remain in charge in emergency situations.
- Know district policies and procedures. Challenge those in conflict with your professional beliefs before they become issues.

Special Issues

▐▌

Autism Spectrum Disorders

It is increasingly clear that schools today are becoming the primary site for detection, intervention, and treatment of a variety of illnesses. This is especially true for mental health issues. No matter how loving or intelligent a child's parents are, this is a painful area. Parents often delay seeking help and find it difficult, if not impossible, to be objective about their own child.

It would be most helpful if there were a clear definition, known cause, and specific treatments for autism. Unfortunately, this information does not yet exist. The body of knowledge is growing, but for now, we must examine what we do know and continue to identify children with autism as early as possible so that they have the best possible prognosis.

In this chapter, you will learn:

1. The definition of autism, along with a history of the disorder, causal theories, and risk factors
2. Classifications of autism, and statistics relating to incidence
3. Signs and symptoms of children with autism
4. Possible comorbid disorders and differential diagnoses
5. School interventions and how to maintain an active role in supporting children with autism, their siblings, and parents

Healthy People 2020 Objective

Maternal, Infant, and Child Health, 29.1

Increase the proportion of children (aged 10–35 months) who have been screened for an Autism Spectrum Disorder (ASD) and other developmental delays from 22.6% in 2007 to 24.9%.

DEFINITION OF AUTISM

Autism is an umbrella term used to describe a group of intricate developmental brain disorders known as pervasive developmental disorders. Autism is a spectrum disorder, which means that all autistic children share some common symptoms but these vary in severity, specificity, and behavior, with overlapping and considerable individual variation. For our purposes, autism spectrum disorder and pervasive developmental disorders are terms that can be used interchangeably.

Autism spectrum disorder cuts across all lines of socioeconomic status, educational background, race, religion, and ethnicity. It is definitely not caused by a lack of maternal nurturing, as previously thought. Most experts would also state that it is not caused by immunizations, though some still cling to this belief.

The Individuals with Disabilities Education Act has identified autism as one of the areas included for services and mandates that every autistic child receive a free, appropriate education in the least restrictive environment. This places an enormous financial burden on the local school districts. It also places an enormous emotional burden on the school nurse.

HISTORY OF AUTISM

In 1938, child psychiatrist Leo Kanner, working out of Johns Hopkins Hospital in Baltimore, Maryland, evaluated 11 children with similarities that he had never seen before. He published his findings in an article entitled "Autistic Disturbances of Affective Contact." Kanner described these children as viewing people as unwelcome intruders in their world, and as being detached and inaccessible. He believed that they lived in a world of their own, where they could not be reached. Kanner used the word *autistic* because he was struck by the children's self-absorption (Bruey, 2004, pp. 30–31).

=== *FAST FACTS in a NUTSHELL*

The word *autism* was also used for people diagnosed with schizophrenia, and many once believed that these were related conditions. Today it is known that the two diseases are separate. Autistic behaviors are easily recognized by the trained observer.

Clinical Snapshot
Mr. and Mrs. Smith have two children. The older daughter is a third-grade student in your school. You have noticed that the preschool-aged younger brother does not maintain eye contact, will not socialize, and engages in repetitive play. He does not attend any preschool program and you are concerned. School nurse Donna suggests to the parents that he be evaluated by the Child Study Team.

CAUSAL THEORIES AND RISK FACTORS

The etiology of autism is still unknown, but it is theorized that, because the disorder involves such a wide spectrum of symptoms, there are most likely many causes. It is believed that an autistic child's brain handles information differently from the way other children's brains do. There are probably a variety of factors that increase the likelihood of a child being in the spectrum of autism, including environmental, biological, and genetic factors. It is generally agreed that autism is a developmental disability and that its basis is organic with a genetic component.

FAST FACTS in a NUTSHELL

Very few diagnoses are feared as much as autism. Helping families of autistic children recognize, accept, and cope with the diagnosis will be the most difficult challenge you meet.

Clinical Snapshot

Once Donna, the school nurse, makes the recommendation for a referral, she must continue to support the parent through the process. Donna may have to deal with resentment on the part of the parent. If a child is found to have behaviors that place him or her within the spectrum, much work will need to be done as early as possible. Early detection and intervention are imperative.

FACTORS INFLUENCING AUTISM

- Genetic predisposition
- A sibling with autism
- Male preponderance
- Presence of another genetic disorder
- Maternal use of certain drugs during pregnancy

AREAS OF CONCERN

Autistic children have deficits in three core areas: social skills, communication, and behavior or interests. Because there is no specific blood test or other diagnostic tool, the diagnosis must be based on behavior, which varies considerably, especially with very young children. In addition, these children may experience fine or gross motor delays or cognitive issues.

Deficit	Behavior
Social skills	Impairment in nonverbal behavior (eye-to-eye contact, facial expressions, gestures)
	Failure to develop appropriate peer relationships; lack of spontaneously sharing enjoyment and ideas
	Lack of emotional reciprocity (acting as if in own world)

(continued)

Deficit	Behavior
Communication	Delay in, or lack of development of, spoken language with no attempt to compensate
	Marked impairment initiating or sustaining a conversation with others who can speak
	Echolalia or pronominal reversal (instead of "I want a drink," it is "Peter wants a drink")
	Lack of varied spontaneous make-believe play or social imitative play that is age appropriate
Behavior or interests	Preoccupation with parts or objects
	Behaviors that are narrow in their focus and repetitive
	Inflexible adherence to routines and rituals
	Stereotyped and repetitive motor mannerisms (hand or finger flapping, complex body movements)

CLASSIFICATIONS OF AUTISM SPECTRUM DISORDERS

There are five recognized types of autism spectrum disorders:

Type	Manifestations
1. Autistic disorder (classic)	Significant language delay
	Social and communication impairment
	Unusual behaviors and interests
	Intellectual disability
	Most common type
2. Asperger's syndrome	Higher functioning form of autism
	Less-pronounced social challenges
	Idiosyncratic social skills and play
	Typical language development
	Average or above-average intellect

(continued)

Type	Manifestations
3. Childhood disintegrative disorder	Typical development for first 2 years
	Regression then occurs between 2 and 4 years
	Developmental behaviors affected: socializing, motor skills, toilet training, use of nonverbal behaviors
	Very rare disorder
4. Rett syndrome	Affects only girls
	Mildly delayed as infants
	By 18 months, have progressive loss of skill in gross motor, language, and social areas
	Growth of head circumference slows
	Difficult gait and balance
	Repetitive hand-wringing and hyperventilating behaviors are common
5. Pervasive developmental disorder: not otherwise specified	This category is considered when there is severe impairment in social skills and verbal communication, but the criteria are not met for another specific area

STATISTICS

It is estimated that in the United States, roughly 1 child of every 110 is considered to be within the autistic spectrum. This includes 1 out of every 70 boys. The ratio is three or four males to one female.

This rate appears to be increasing by 10% to 17% annually. The reason for this dramatic increase is not clear, but most would agree that there are now better means of detection and the definition of autism has been broadened to include many additional conditions. Regardless of the cause, there are more children with autism than with cancer, diabetes, and AIDS combined (Autism Speaks, 2010).

Most parents recall starting to be concerned when the child is around 1 year of age. Severe problems can be noted earlier, whereas some children may not demonstrate deficits until closer to 2 years. Children's development may appear to be age appropriate until 18 to 24 months and then cease to progress.

Usually, autism is diagnosed around age 3 and will be a lifelong condition. Early signs to watch for include the following:

- Not responding to name by 12 months
- Not pointing to objects of interest by 14 months
- Not playing pretend games by 18 months
- Avoiding eye contact
- Difficulty understanding feelings, their own or others
- Delayed speech and language skills
- Echolalia
- Spinning, rocking, and flapping
- Sensory issues (Centers for Disease Control and Prevention, 2006)

THE FAMILY

As with all other major health issues, the family of an autistic child is significantly affected. Parents often go through stages of denial, fear, anger, and panic, and their concerns are indeed warranted. At best, they must be prepared for a lifetime of challenges with the very real possibility that their child may never be fully independent. The school nurse will play an important role as parents go through the process of acceptance of their child's special needs. The school nurse can be of even greater help with any siblings.

Be mindful of the impact this diagnosis has on siblings. Parents tend to focus on the child with the greatest needs and can unintentionally neglect the other children. The family may experience financial difficulties if one parents needs to stay at home to be available for physician visits and various therapies. Stress may cause marital unrest and even further pain for the other children. Seek out these siblings and support their needs as well.

COMORBID DISORDERS

A number of disorders are associated with autism spectrum disorder. These disorders can overlap. Alone, they cannot be diagnostic of autism; however, the school nurse needs to be mindful of the possibility of their presence.

Some Comorbid Disorders Associated With Autism

- Seizures
- Immune system dysfunction
- Hyperactivity
- Anxiety
- Gastrointestinal disorders
- Allergies
- Obsessive behaviors
- Depression

DIFFERENTIAL DIAGNOSES

Often, children with autism have more than one problem. Multiple issues can become apparent and take various forms and different combinations. One issue can easily exacerbate another, so each must be addressed and handled appropriately.

The school nurse needs to be aware that when a diagnosis of autism spectrum disorder has been made, the following conditions must be considered, as well, to determine their possible influence on the child's behavior:

- Speech and language disorders; aphasia
- Social phobia
- Central auditory processing disorder
- Mentally challenged
- Oppositional defiant disorder
- Hearing impairment
- Chromosomal or metabolic disorders

- Attention deficit disorder
- Learning disability
- Sensory integration dysfunction
- Anxiety; obsessive–compulsive disorder
- Tourette syndrome
- Depression
- Bipolar disorder

SCHOOL INTERVENTIONS

Schools can take a number of steps to help children with autism.

- Early detection
  - Preschool programs have afforded professionals the opportunity to see children at younger ages. This allows us to detect problems and intervene early. The sooner a child is diagnosed and treated, the better the outcome will be.
  - Siblings of diagnosed children must be assessed as early as possible because they may also have a genetic component predisposing them to autism.
- Child Study Team involvement
  - A team approach is needed for speech, occupational, and physical therapy. Children who need such therapy, if necessary, are placed in a self-contained classroom.
  - Behavior modification, communication therapy, and social skills development are essential.
- Intervention strategies
  - The classroom environment must be structured.
  - The teacher must be educated about the specific needs of the autistic child.
  - The teacher should develop consistent, predictable routines and schedules.
  - The teacher should determine the child's learning style and present new information appropriately.
  - Sensory stimulation, such as loud noises, should be limited.
  - Peer mentoring and small-group activities with mainstream students should be encouraged.
  - Positive reinforcement should be used as much as possible.

FAST FACTS in a NUTSHELL

Before attempting to help families of children with autism, find out what they know and have already been told. Clarify misconceptions and build on the strengths of the child.

Clinical Snapshot

Mr. and Mrs. Smith have accepted that their son is within the autism spectrum. Mrs. Smith frequently calls to speak with Donna, the school nurse, and asks advice. Donna needs to be careful with what she shares. She needs to check to see what parents have previously been told by the physician and other members of the Child Study Team and to support her colleagues. If she vehemently disagrees with what a parent has been told, she needs to go back to the source for clarification and have them discuss it with the parent.

ROLE OF THE SCHOOL NURSE IN HELPING CHILDREN WITH AUTISM AND THEIR FAMILIES

- Encourage the development of and attendance in preschool programs in your district to facilitate early detection.
- Be alert for signs and symptoms of autism spectrum disorder in children, especially if one sibling has already been diagnosed.
- Actively participate in Intervention and Referral Services or Child Study Team meetings, or both, to identify and plan the program for these children.
- In working with the parents, attempt to determine their level of knowledge, perspective, and coping skills regarding their child's diagnosis. Build on this information.
- Prepare the medical component for the Individualized Education Plan.
- Prepare the Individualized Healthcare Plan, 504 Accommodation Plan, or Emergency Care Plan, as needed.
- Be mindful that comorbid diseases and differential diagnoses are possible.
- Serve as a health resource and liaison for staff, family, and student.
- Consider referral to outside community agencies when warranted.

12

Adolescent Sexuality and Mental Health Issues

Adolescence marks the passage from child to adult. It is considered the most crucial stage in human lives. One's physical appearance changes dramatically, and the brain evolves further. Adolescents have the opportunity to begin to prioritize responsibilities so they can make good decisions and become fully functioning, productive adults.

Each child goes through many rapid changes in growth—physically, socially, emotionally, and intellectually—as he or she begins to develop more advanced thinking skills in preparation for adulthood. The fact that all these changes take place in a relatively short period of time causes confusion and turbulence for adolescents and all who surround them.

In this chapter, you will learn:

1. How the brain develops
2. The stages of adolescence
3. The physical and mental changes common to all adolescents
4. Factors that influence adolescents
5. Various mental disorders and issues affecting today's adolescents
6. Sexual health disorders and issues of today's adolescents
7. Strategies the school nurse can use to help identify and treat adolescents experiencing extreme difficulty

THE RAPIDLY CHANGING BODY AND BRAIN

Physiologically, adolescence presents many unique challenges as compared with other growth periods. Physical and mental disturbances increase in proportion to these changes. As a child begins to mature, he or she shows sexual interest, seeks autonomy, is susceptible to growing peer influence, and is expected to achieve academic success. These multiple interchanging influences can cause overwhelming stress, which will have an impact on the educational process. An unhappy, insecure child cannot learn. Basic needs for belonging and acceptance must be met first.

FAST FACTS in a NUTSHELL

Today we recognize that there are significant changes as the brain develops. These changes account for the adolescent's unpredictable behavior.

Clinical Snapshot

Josh is sent to sit with you to *cool off*. He refused to cooperate in math class and was rude to his teacher. You sit next to this now-sweet 14-year-old and ask what the problem was. Josh tries to explain his poor behavior but seems generally confused himself. School nurse Lisa is constantly amazed by the inconsistencies apparent in teens.

These inconsistencies are seen both between teens and day to day within individual teens. It is not uncommon for a teen to behave appropriately in one setting and quite irrationally in another.

Today's effective diagnostic tools and research allow us to begin to understand the rapid changes in function as the brain continues to mature during adolescence. Brain development progresses from the posterior to the frontal lobes. This latter area, known as the prefrontal cortex, is the portion designated for planning and recognizing consequences. It is the last part of the brain to develop.

The prefrontal cortex communicates with the rest of the brain through connections called synapses. A tremendous growth in synapses occurs during adolescence. Because children mature at different rates, it is easy to understand why some have more difficulty during this phase of development. Their brains have not yet advanced in the area needed for decision making (Edmonds, 2012).

Adolescence is also a time when there is an opportunity to establish the skills and values needed for adult life. Most children do just that and find their way with minimal issues. Unfortunately, we most often hear about the negative aspects and behaviors of adolescents. For some, the path to full, productive, adult potential may have obstacles such as illness, frequent moves, the death of a loved one, or a family financial crisis. Everyday problems can turn into large ones or into complex disorders that cloud the path and add to the stress that a child is experiencing.

The school nurse's role is to recognize the struggling students, and to clear and illuminate the path as we guide them along. If the path is totally blocked, a student will need an entirely different approach. Sometimes, the alternate path will also have obstacles. A student can be misdiagnosed, experience ineffective treatment, have additional issues that were overlooked, or have parents who are reluctant to seek help altogether. Even the best-educated, loving parent can fail to recognize or accept the seriousness of an adolescent's problems.

The goal, of course, is to recognize a lost child early and provide him or her with a safe, accepting path to adulthood. It is essential to identify an obstacle before it becomes an overwhelming disorder. Once the school nurse helps such a child find the correct path, it can lead to full, productive, adult behavior, and the student can reach his or her full potential.

Other chapters in this book address important issues that affect adolescents, including obesity, substance abuse, and bullying.

=== *FAST FACTS in a NUTSHELL*

Adolescence commences around 10 years and ends between 18 and 24 years. Some experts divide adolescence into stages: early—10 to 13 years; middle—14 to 17; and late—18 to 20 years.

Clinical Snapshot

Twelve-year-old Keisha and her younger brother are in the sole custody of her dad. Mother is incarcerated with little chance of obtaining freedom. Aware of this, school nurse Lisa speaks with Keisha's dad and, with his permission, offer to talk privately with her about menstruation and other anticipated bodily changes.

As students progress from one stage to another, there can be confusion. In school, they are surrounded by peers dealing with their own unrest while at home they may be alone in going through this tumultuous time. When there is little or no support at home, the school nurse can be available to help.

STAGES OF ADOLESCENCE

Stage	Age	Typical Behaviors
Early	10–13	Thinks in concrete terms; can categorize thoughts into usable forms; little consideration of long-term consequences
		Behavior may be rebellious, defiant of adult authority
		Lacks self-esteem
		Attempts to seek own identity; begins to question family values
		Influenced significantly by peers; uses peer-group "language"; adopts peer-group clothing style
Middle	14–17	Thinking is more abstract; begins to think of, and be concerned about, long-term consequences
		Increasing interest in sex
		Continues to develop definition of self, especially with intimate relationships; concerns over physical and sexual attractiveness
		May experiment with drugs (cigarettes, alcohol, marijuana) and sex
		Moodiness
		Seeks greater independence from family; may complain that family interferes; seeks privacy from family
		Tests rules and behavioral limits
Late	18–20	Begins to make independent choices
		Seeks additional responsibilities
		Establishes relationship with a significant other
		Finds employment or goes to college

Adapted from Selekman (2006, p. 378); Scudder (2006, p. 1319); Garber (2010, p. 58, 73); and American Academy of Child and Adolescent Psychiatry (2004).

ADOLESCENT CHANGES

Physical Maturity

Puberty begins during early adolescence and progresses systematically for both boys and girls. Each child goes through the various stages according to his or her own pattern. Thus, children of the same grade and age can appear quite different in terms of physical maturation. This can cause some to have a poor body image and lower self-esteem.

Anticipated Appearance and Behaviors

- Tremendous physical growth
- Appearance of secondary sex characteristics

Behaviors That Are Cause for Concern

- Physical confrontations
- Bullying

Sexual Interest

Adolescence is the time when children begin to show interest in sexual issues and partners. Early experiences consist mostly of thoughts that are not acted upon. During the middle and late adolescent stages, young people seek their sexual identity and begin to form meaningful relationships.

Anticipated Appearance and Behaviors

- Greater interest in sexual issues
- Girls—breast and hip changes; Boys—growth in penis and testicles, occurrence of wet dreams

Behaviors That Are Cause for Concern

- Promiscuity
- Unprotected sex

Autonomy

Adolescents urgently seek to be their own person. A close, strong family bond helps to ground them for future changes and decision making, but separation is clearly a healthy behavior.

Anticipated Appearance or Behaviors

- Questioning adult decisions
- Recognition that parents and teachers are fallible

Behaviors That Are Cause for Concern

- Repeated rule and limit testing
- Withdrawal from family
- School truancy and phobias

Peer Relations

Peer relations are important at this time. Most adolescents care more about what friends think than about what parents think. This is normal and to be expected. During late adolescence, young people begin to seek that one special partner.

Anticipated Appearance or Behaviors

- Desire to be popular with peers
- Self-involvement

Behaviors That Are Cause for Concern

- Partnerships with gangs
- Weapon possession
- Illegal drug use
- Talk of suicide
- Self-injury
- Depression

FACTORS INFLUENCING ADOLESCENCE

There are four factors that significantly influence the adolescent in his or her journey toward adulthood.

1. Biological influences: Hormones have a significant impact on physical, emotional, and psychological changes as a child goes

Adolescent issues is an area on which experts are just beginning to focus. It is felt that unrecognized problems at this age can lead to serious adult problems in later years.

Clinical Snapshot

David's family moved numerous times during his high school years. As soon as he formed friendships, his dad received another transfer. School nurse Lisa notes that David has difficulty establishing peer relationships, is emotionally distant, and appears unhappy. She points this out to his teachers and asks them to join you in monitoring David's socialization. This is discussed at the parent–teacher conference so David's parents are aware of the possible long-term effects on their child.

through puberty. The appearance of secondary sex characteristics, such as female breast development and male facial hair, can threaten self-image. Some adolescents enjoy their new, grown-up appearances, whereas others become self-conscious and awkward.

2. Cognitive influences: Adolescents begin to think more rationally. They begin to think in hypothetical terms that extend beyond the "here and now." They work hard to develop their own identities and, ideally, healthy self-esteem.

3. Emotional influences: Adolescents start to develop the ability to understand and control their emotions. They begin to comprehend relationships in a mature way and think things through from different perspectives. Yet, they remain neither child nor adult.

4. Social influences: Adolescents tend to focus all their interest on peers and begin to develop romantic relationships. They seek more privacy from family members and want their own identities. They begin to acquire rights: to drive, to earn money, to vote, and so on. Along with these rights come added responsibilities: home obligations, academic expectations, assistance to younger siblings, contributions to home finances.

Tweens

Tweens are a newly identified group of children between ages 8 and 11 years who are entering the adolescent stage of development.

Advertisers named this group of children and now target specific clothing and personal items to this market. Technology plays a significant part in enhancing this effort. Some educators and parents fear that this will lead to exposure to sexual experiences before some children are ready for them. Of course, most parents prefer that their children remain children as long as possible.

MENTAL HEALTH DISORDERS AND ISSUES

The issues described below are commonly diagnosed during adolescence. If unrecognized or left untreated, they can lead to school failure and tremendous suffering for the student and his or her family. It is not the responsibility of the school nurse to diagnose these disorders. Rather, the nurse's role is to understand their prevalence in adolescents, observe for early signs and symptoms, and make referrals immediately when necessary. Frequently, following a referral, counseling will be recommended or medication will be prescribed, or both.

Isolation

Belonging to a group and community is a fundamental need of all people. A student who frequently moves or is not accepted by peers must be closely observed. Signs and symptoms of isolation include:

- Refusal to participate in group activities
- Sudden, dramatic change in appearance
- Talk of suicide
- Talk or evidence of self-harm
- Peers expressing concern

Anxiety

Anxiety is a manifestation of stress and fear that has no clear cause. Signs and symptoms include:

- Difficulty breathing
- Nausea
- Tachycardia

- Persistent negative thoughts
- Fears that interfere with activities

Eating Disorders

Adolescents may become obsessed with looking thin to such an extreme that they become ill. The two most common eating disorders are bulimia nervosa and anorexia nervosa.

Bulimia Nervosa

Signs and symptoms of bulimia include:

- Binging: eating a large amount of food in a short period of time
- Purging: forcing oneself to vomit

Anorexia Nervosa

Signs and symptoms of anorexia include:

- Severe dieting
- Excessive exercise
- Abuse of laxatives

Obsessive–Compulsive Disorders

Persons with these disorders experience repetitive, unwanted thoughts that become uncontrollable, repetitive behaviors. Signs and symptoms include:

- Fear of germs
- Fear of things being out of order
- Repetitive counting, tapping, words, or phrases

Phobias

Phobias are excessive, unreasonable fears in response to objects or events. They are usually triggered by some event. Signs and symptoms of phobias include:

- Overwhelming anxiety or panic
- A need to escape
- Knowledge of overreaction but powerless to control self

Mood Disorders (Affective Disorders)

Everyone is capable of experiencing a wide range of moods, and irritability is common. Mood disorders are diagnosed when extremes of mood or irritability interfere with a student's ability to perform the activities of daily life. Signs and symptoms include:

- Depression
- Excessive fatigue
- Loss of appetite

Suicide

Suicide is rare in early adolescence but becomes more common in later stages of adolescence. It remains a hidden problem and is the third leading cause of death among adolescents aged 10 to 19 years. Signs and symptoms of suicidal potential include:

- Familial history of suicide or violence
- Previous attempt
- Depression

Self-Injury Disorders

Adolescents may experience such extreme internal pain or anger that they attempt to harm themselves by cutting or undergoing excessive tattooing. Signs and symptoms of self-injury include:

- Fresh, unexplained cuts or bruises
- Wearing long sleeves in very warm weather
- Emotional instability

Healthy People 2020 Objective

Mental Health and Mental Disorders, 4.1

Reduce the proportion of adolescents aged 12 to 17 years who experience major depressive episodes (MDEs) from 8.3% in 2008 to 7.4%.

Sexual Orientation

Sexuality is part of the normal development of a person's identity. Adolescents frequently are fearful about their gender identity. This fear is warranted because of continuing discrimination against homosexual, bisexual, and transgender people.

=====================*FAST FACTS in a NUTSHELL*

Sexuality should be thought of as occurring on a continuum with heterosexuality at one end and homosexuality at the other. All people are at different points on that continuum.

Clinical Snapshot

Matthew is a frail, gentle ninth grader who is frequently tormented by groups of his peers, who call him names and harass him in the hallways. In an anonymous question box, he asks the school nurse, Lisa, how he will know if he is gay.

One response might be to explain that sexuality is not a choice but a combination of genetic, hormonal, and environmental factors. Explain that there is no way that you or anyone else can tell if Matthew is gay at this age, but when he is older, it will be clearer. Assure him that he is perfect just the way he is. For now, if the subject of homosexuality, or any other topic, is really troubling him, you can arrange for Matthew to talk privately with a counselor about his feelings.

Risky Behaviors

Young adolescents have not mastered the ability to think in the long term, so they tend to be involved with behaviors that can cause immediate and long-term harm. Drinking, driving, and drug use are significant concerns during adolescence.

Teen Parenting

In recent years, there has been progress in reducing the number of teen pregnancies; however, a significant number of teens still become pregnant. This is a crisis for the adolescent mother and father, and their families. Many teens choose to abort, but many others carry and keep their babies while remaining in school. Children rarely make good parents, and a baby born to teen parents will likely suffer despite the best intentions of the parents.

Sexually Transmitted Diseases

The great majority of those who contract sexually transmitted diseases (STDs) are younger than 25 years of age. In addition, adolescents are at high risk for reinfection because they frequently do not notify partners or seek prompt treatment. Despite the availability of drug therapy, HIV infection carries a death threat. Chlamydia, gonorrhea, and pelvic inflammatory disease are the most common STDs diagnosed among adolescents.

FAST FACTS in a NUTSHELL

Sexuality is an area where discretion is a priority. Do not gossip with colleagues. Make sure files are secure, and document only what you must according to district policy. We carry a tremendous responsibility for students who have mental health and sexuality issues and are just a little different. Watch the quiet ones. No one hears their voices until it is too late.

Clinical Snapshot

Amanda is a newly enrolled ninth grader. She appears depressed, isolates herself, and refuses overtures from you and her peers to participate in school functions. School nurse Lisa notices that she wears long sleeves even in warm weather and are concerned she might be cutting. Lisa speaks with her and asks her if she has ever considered hurting herself. Lisa asks Amanda if she can see her arms and will refer immediately for psychiatric evaluation if scars are seen or she expresses suicidal thoughts. Lisa will continue to invite her to join the school health club or find tasks for her to do in your office. Lisa will gradually help her integrate into the school community while affording her a warm place to visit and find acceptance.

ROLE OF SCHOOL NURSES IN ADOLESCENT SEXUALITY AND MENTAL HEALTH ISSUES

- Continue to listen and be approachable to all students.
- Empower students with education to help them make appropriate decisions.
- Remain connected to the school and community.
- Try to involve all students in some group activity.
- Provide support within the school, especially if it is lacking at home.
- When planning to intervene, allow the adolescent to be part of the plan.
- Appreciate the importance of each student's problem, whether it is a breakup with a boyfriend or girlfriend, difficulties with peers, teasing, bullying, and so on.
- Identify any lost, unhappy children and provide them with support.
- Check the curriculum and make sure sex education includes information about abstinence, the use of condoms, teen parenting, and the prevention of STDs.

13

Childhood Obesity

The fastest growing epidemic in our country is obesity, affecting all ages with devastating short- and long-term complications. Childhood obesity causes serious risk factors for many major illnesses and unprecedented financial and social costs to our nation. Some health professionals feel that the schools have contributed to the problem with fat- and sugar-laden school lunches, celebrations, vending machine offerings, bake sales, and lack of recess or physical education during the school day. Legislation to combat the rise of obesity has been proposed and implemented to support school districts in offering healthier food choices and more opportunities for physical activity. Today's statistics on obesity are truly alarming. This epidemic requires immediate attention if we are to stem this public health crisis.

The school nurse has the important role of assessing and managing overweight and obese children in the school setting, as well as implementing prevention programs. Part of our task is to look closely at obese students and staff members and recognize the depth of their suffering.

In this chapter, you will learn:

1. The scope of the childhood obesity crisis
2. How to identify children who are obese and overweight

3. Causes of obesity, and the emotional components of food
4. Consequences of obesity
5. Preventive programs and support that can be initiated within the school

SCOPE OF THE CHILDHOOD OBESITY CRISIS

According to the Centers for Disease Control and Prevention (CDC, 2008), the prevalence of overweight children in the United States has reached alarming levels. Statistics clearly show that childhood obesity has more than tripled in the past 30 years. The rate of obesity for children aged 6 to 11 years increased from 6.5% in 1980 to 19.6% in 2008. Adolescents aged 12 to 19 years showed a similar increase, from 5% to 18%. Sadly, it appears that childhood obesity is a trend that will continue growing unless steps are immediately taken to get it under control.

Healthy People 2020 Objectives

Nutrition and Weight Status, 10.3

Reduce the proportion of children and adolescents aged 12 to 19 years who are considered obese from 17.9% to 16.1%.

Physical Activity, 4.1–4.3

Increase the proportion of the nation's public and private schools that require daily physical education for all students:

Elementary—from 3.8% in 2006 to 4.2%

Middle—from 7.8% in 2006 to 8.6%

High—from 2.1% in 2006 to 2.3%

Physical Activity, 6.2

Increase the proportion of school districts that require regularly scheduled elementary school recess from 57.1% in 2006 to 62.8%.

IDENTIFYING OVERWEIGHT OR OBESE CHILDREN

When a person is overweight or obese, there is an excess of body fat. The person is taking in more calories than his or her level of activity requires. Excess calories are stored as fat in the body. If overconsumption of calories is persistent, fat accumulates, causing weight gain.

================================ *FAST FACTS in a NUTSHELL*

Obese children may be rejected by their peers and will cope by simply eating more. Society's attitude toward these individuals is probably the one type of prejudice still tolerated within schools, communities, and the nation itself.

Clinical Snapshot

Consuela is a 12-year old sixth-grade student, who was adopted at birth from Central America. She is 62 inches tall, weighs 230 pounds, is hypertensive (BP of 160/100), and has a BMI over 95%. Untidy and socially isolated, she is a very unhappy young girl. Previous attempts by the school nurse, Mary Ellen, to communicate concern to the parents proved unsuccessful and produced angry accusations of intrusiveness. As graduation to middle school approached, Consuela became even heavier and developed school phobia, refusing most days to get out of bed. Mom has now asked for help.

A problem must be acknowledged before change can take place. The school nurse is now in a position to help this family. Consuela should be referred for a comprehensive physical examination, and an Individualized Healthcare Plan should be developed.

The first step in determining whether a child is overweight or obese is to calculate his or her body mass index (BMI). This is the quickest and easiest screening tool. School nurses check students' height and weight annually. From these numbers, the BMI of each student can be calculated. BMI is determined by using the following formula (CDC, 2014a):

$$\text{weight (lb)}/[\text{height (in)}]^2 \times 703$$

The number obtained is then referenced on the CDC's BMI-for-age growth charts for girls and boys. *See Appendix F for BMI graphs for boys and girls.* The acceptable amount of body fat changes with age and differs for boys and girls. Where a child's BMI falls on the graph determines the level of concern for the child:

- Underweight: Less than the 5th percentile
- Healthy weight: 5th percentile to less than the 85th percentile
- Overweight: 85th percentile to less than the 95th percentile
- Obese: Equal to or greater than the 95th percentile
- For the purposes of this chapter, the terms *obesity* and *overweight* are used interchangeably.

CAUSES OF CHILDHOOD OBESITY

As noted by Bellows and Moore (March, 2013), many variables can cause obesity, including those listed in the following sections. Frequently, these variables interact to create even greater problems for obese children.

Genetics

Certain people are simply more susceptible to weight gain. We can see clearly that obesity runs in families. Parental obesity is a strong predictor for child obesity.

Behavior

Some behaviors contribute to weight gain. These include eating an unhealthful diet, engaging in limited physical activities, and having a sedentary lifestyle.

Diet

- Reliance on fast foods
- Preference for high-sugar snacks and drinks
- Use of large portion sizes
- Use of food as a reward
- Few meals eaten with family

Activities

- Excessive screen time (e.g., watching television, computer, video games)
- Little or no participation in sports
- Fewer children walking to and from school

Lifestyle

- Sedentary lifestyle
- Frequent snacking on junk foods

Environment

The home and school setting may both contribute to obesity. Children with working parents may be told to wait for their parents at the public library or to go directly home, lock the door, and stay inside until a parent gets home. They may not be permitted to play outside unsupervised for safety reasons. This contributes to boredom, snacking, and lack of physical activity.

Sociodemographics

Families with low-income levels may not be able to provide their children with healthful choices such as fresh fruits and vegetables.

EMOTIONAL COMPONENTS OF FOOD

Rimm (2004) explained that food means different things to different people. To understand the meanings that food may have for an obese child, consider the following emotional components.

Food Is Love

- Babies are conditioned to equate food with love. If an infant cries or is cranky, we feed him or her. We offer milk, cookies, juice, cereal, or whatever it takes to make the baby stop crying.
- Therefore, if food is love, does the withdrawal of food mean the baby is not loved?

Food Is Health

- We consider a chubby baby to be healthy. Small children are encouraged to eat so they grow "strong and healthy."
- If we feed them less, does that mean they are not healthy?

Food Is Celebration

- Every time people of all cultures gather in joy, we celebrate with food. This means that birthdays, holidays, a new job, graduation, wedding, and so on all justify eating. The more important the occasion, the more elaborate the food.
- If we eat less rich food, does the occasion have less significance?

Food Is Basic

- We simply love to eat! It satisfies our basic need for nourishment and gives us great pleasure. Most Americans can afford to eat as much and as often as they wish, and that is exactly what we do.
- So, because we can afford food, why can't we eat what we want?

Food Is Social Status

- Many important interviews and celebrations are held at expensive restaurants. Guests are entertained lavishly at dinners in four- and five-star restaurants with elite clientele who can afford the best.
- Do we not deserve this too?

Food Is Power

- Some children control the dinner table by refusing to eat or by gorging themselves. They use food to manipulate their parents into bribing them: "Just finish what is on your plate and then you can have a present."
- Isn't it important to get the child to eat using any means possible?

- Parents rejoice when the pediatrician announces that their child is thriving and has attained high growth and weight percentages. At some point, however, this can become a problem for parents who realize that their child is becoming obese.
- Why can't we be complacent in this situation?

CONSEQUENCES OF OBESITY

The physical and psychosocial consequences of childhood obesity are frightening, both in the short term and the long term.

Physical Consequences	Duration of Impact
Adult obesity	Long term
Gallbladder disease	Long term
Heart disease and hypertension	Long and short term
Hyperlipidemia	Long term
Diabetes mellitus type 2	Long term
Early sexual maturation	Short term
Asthma	Long and short term
Sleep disturbances (e.g., apnea)	Long and short term
Musculoskeletal diseases	Long term
Depression	Long and short term
Social ineptness	Long and short term
Victim of bullying	Long and short term
Poor body image	Long and short term
Reduced quality of life	Long and short term
Low academic achievement	Long and short term
Poor school attendance	Short term

Each state develops its own curriculum content standards. These address the subject to be taught, and at what grade level, as well as strategies to help students develop skills to reduce high-risk health-related behaviors. The curriculum standards are vaguely written, allowing teachers to individualize lessons to meet the needs of the student and class. If obesity is prevalent in a particular class, lessons should be focused accordingly.

Clinical Snapshot

When school nurse Mary Ellen reviewed the entire class BMI statistics, she noted that Consuela was not the only obese child in her class. Therefore, a broader approach needed to be taken. Mary Ellen sat down with the class room teacher and altered the health curriculum to focus more on proper food intake and the importance of exercise.

SCHOOL INITIATIVES TO PREVENT CHILDHOOD OBESITY

Childhood obesity is best addressed by using each of the eight components of the coordinated school health program introduced in Chapter 1.

1. *Comprehensive school health program:* In this organized, sequential K–12 plan for delivering information, students are given factual information about diet and diseases throughout their school experience. This helps them make wise health decisions based on factual information.
2. *Physical education:* This component is a planned, sequential K–12 curriculum that provides cognitive content and experiences in a variety of activities, including basic movement skills, physical fitness, rhythm and dance, and individual and team sports. This component is especially important for students who are not physically active outside of school.
3. *School health services:* These services include the school nurse's role in measuring each student's height and weight to determine his or her BMI. This is how overweight children are identified, and steps to help them are initiated.
4. *Nutrition services:* These include services that provide students with nutritionally balanced, varied meals and healthful snacks

in an atmosphere that promotes social interaction. All students should have only nutritious choices available.

5. *Counseling, psychological, and social services:* These are services that offer broad-based individual and group assessments, interventions, and referrals that attend to the mental, emotional, and social needs of students. Obese students may need more services than can be offered at school. Referrals to appropriate outside agencies may be warranted.

6. *Healthful and safe school environment:* A healthful and safe school environment is one that is free of prejudice against people who are obese and supports every person's need for acceptance and belonging within the school community.

7. *Health promotion for staff:* Health promotion programs such as health screenings, assessments, health education, and physical activities are important for the wellness and morale of staff. Teachers must be well themselves before they can effectively teach students.

8. *Parent/family and community involvement:* Schools need to partner with parents and community groups to address the needs of obese students. Obesity is often a problem for siblings and parents as well, and informed, involved parents can greatly help obese children. Often, community agencies sponsor health-related activities in which these children can participate.

FAST FACTS in a NUTSHELL

When talking with the family of an obese child, the topic of weight must be handled sensitively. Parents may be offended and feel you are intruding. Obesity may very well be only a symptom of a greater problem. Tread lightly in this area as parents may be defensive. Recognize and seek professional help for morbidly obese children or adults.

Clinical Snapshot

Consuela's mom immediately became defensive when she received the referral letter that her daughter brought home the day after school nurse Mary Ellen conducted height and weight screenings at school. A better approach might have been for Mary Ellen to make a phone call letting the mother know that she would be getting the BMI referral in the mail shortly. An explanation of school policy and your sincere concern may soften a parent's irate reaction.

ROLE OF SCHOOL NURSES IN SUPPORTING THOSE WHO ARE OVERWEIGHT

- Check each student's, height, weight, and BMI annually and make referrals as necessary.
- Organize a group of concerned students, staff, and parents to work with you on preventive programs such as health clubs, walking groups, weight monitoring, and so on.
- Educate students, parents, and staff about the immediate and long-term effects of childhood obesity.
- Create opportunities for the use of school gyms, weight rooms, and playground areas outside of school hours.
- Support local, state, and federal obesity prevention programs.
- Address the issues of healthful diets and exercise through the comprehensive school health curriculum.
- Assess the school's current health policy and procedures. Seek to update and improve them as necessary.
- Evaluate and implement changes in school lunch and party policies.
- Evaluate and implement changes in food catering menus and vending machine offerings.
- Be part of community efforts outside of school to enhance healthful lifestyles.
- Develop 504 or Individualized Healthcare Plans as needed for obese students and staff.
- Encourage such events as "Health Food Sales" or "Salad Days" as fundraisers instead of candy sales.
- Encourage outdoor play at recess, gym, and lunchtimes.
- Celebrate the individual's strengths. Look at the total child.
- In providing health counseling, attempt to coach, rather than judge.
- Focus on lifestyle changes rather than diet alone.
- Be a role model.

14

Drug Use

Ask any school nurse what the school district's substance abuse policy is, and you will be impressed: she will recite it verbatim. She will also know how to identify students who might be using drugs, as well as the correct form to use in reporting related observations.

Ask that same school nurse what she and her school district do to identify those who are **at risk** for drug use, and there will be stunned silence. When the nurse eventually recovers the ability to speak, she will most likely offer to get back to you with the information.

Note that, in this chapter, information relevant to students also applies to staff members. Regarding substance abuse, the school nurse is the teacher, and the needs of both adults and students are the same in terms of requiring early detection, treatment, and support.

Confidentiality is crucial for all, although the legal parameters are different for minor children.

In this chapter, you will learn:

1. The definition of drug abuse
2. The levels of school and district drug education programs
3. Risk factors and protective factors that influence students
4. How to develop a prevention plan for those at risk for drug use, and strategies to help those who are already dependent

DEFINITION

Drug Use and Abuse

A drug is a chemical substance that affects the way the body or mind functions. Drugs can treat diseases, promote health, or make a person ill, depending on how they are used. The inappropriate use of any drug, under any circumstances, is considered abuse.

FAST FACTS in a NUTSHELL

Drugs that can cause dependence are restricted by age (e.g., tobacco and alcohol), availability (e.g., prescription pain medication), or laws (e.g., marijuana and cocaine).

Clinical Snapshot

School nurse Helen is becoming increasingly concerned about a senior student, David. He attendance is poor and he is a social isolate. After noting David's discomfort during a class on addiction he reveals that his parents have a variety of common ailments and, therefore, a medicine cabinet stocked with numerous medications for their use. David began abusing drugs at age 12, with his parents completely unaware that he was slowly, systematically helping himself to their medications and becoming increasingly addicted.

Drug abuse and the concerns of today are quite different from those of the past. More over-the-counter and prescription drugs are being used by younger children (Centers for Disease Control and Prevention, 2010). Gateway drugs such as alcohol and tobacco are being tried by children as young as 9 or 10 years of age. At such early ages, addiction is more likely and costly in terms of both monetary funds and academic performance. The emotional toll is even more devastating. Large-scale national and state programs have not made the hoped-for impact of changing behavior.

Healthy People 2020 Objectives
Substance Abuse, 19.5

Reduce the past-year nonmedical use of any psychotherapeutic drug (including pain relievers, tranquilizers, stimulants, and sedatives) by person aged 12 years and older from 6.1% in 2008 to 5.5%.

TYPES OF PROGRAMS

To best meet the drug education needs of all students, every school and district should have three levels of programs.

Level One: Preventive (For All Students)

Schools today must teach health education as part of the required content areas for learning. The curriculum, learning objectives, and lesson plans are written by the classroom teacher to address the specific drug education needs of the learners. The health teacher must first understand what drugs are commonly used by the students in his or her classes and focus on these.

Level Two: Preventive (For High-Risk Students)

Know your students. Recognize the students at risk and the times that create extreme stress in their lives, and be available. Approach these students, acknowledge the difficult time they are having, and ask that they let you know if they need help. Check resources within the school system. If necessary, offer to investigate available community programs that work with high-risk students and provide prevention strategies to avoid experimenting with drugs or alcohol and halt the progression into drug dependence. This is the area in which much can be done and the school nurse can be most effective.

Level Three: Intervention (For Those Already Drug Dependent)

Once a person is diagnosed and involved in a treatment plan, the school nurse can be invaluable in offering support to the student and his or her family once they return to school. Know what the student's follow-up plan entails and seek to be part of it.

Parental attitudes toward drug use can be a major obstacle. Be aware of what is acceptable at home before you attempt to work with the student. You may need to begin by educating the parent.

🔘 Clinical Snapshot

David Johnson is 17, the youngest of three children. His older siblings attended prestigious universities and are successful and productive. The liquor cabinet in his home has always been left open and available to him, as it was to his brothers. His parents expect that he will drink with his friends, both at home and away from home. They ask only that he not drive while intoxicated. The Johnsons permit other underaged children to drink in their home as well and are in denial that any harm could come from this arrangement. Helen is aware that some of this drinking is occurring at lunchtime and informs the parents that she will follow the school policy on reporting suspicion of alcohol use. She works with her school's parent group to conduct educational programs in an attempt to change attitudes toward underage drinking.

PREVENTIVE APPROACH FOR ALL STUDENTS

A preventive approach is effective for the vast number of students. Teachers are highly qualified to provide factual, necessary information and guide students to make prudent choices.

Role of School Nurses in the Preventive Approach for All Students

- Be a role model for healthful habits.
- Stay current with information on drug use in your school and community.
- Check on what is presently taught in the classrooms.
- Help write the health curriculum.
- Make time in your busy schedule to teach, both in the classroom and one-on-one.

- Partner with community organizations such as the parent–teacher association (PTA) and the police (Drug Abuse Resistance Education) to offer special learning opportunities for students.
- Know your district's policies and procedures for suspected drug abuse. If you disagree, question and seek change *before* any incidents occur.

PREVENTIVE PROGRAMS FOR HIGH-RISK STUDENTS

A health education program such as that outlined earlier is sufficient for most students. However, the greatest concern is for students with risk factors for substance use. Students with one or more of the following characteristics are more likely than others to abuse drugs.

Risk Factors

- Aggressive behavior at a young age
- Unrest within the family
- Family members or close peers who abuse drugs
- Low income levels
- Mentally challenged
- Drug availability
- Low self-esteem
- Social ineptness

Students who are less likely to abuse drugs have what are called protective factors.

Protective Factors

- Stable family life
- Adequate income level
- Community and school support
- Good social skills
- Disciplined lifestyle
- Confidence
- Resistance skills
- Academic achievement

The Goal

According to the National Institute on Drug Abuse (2010, p. 7), the goal of preventive programs for students with risk factors is to change the balance of risk factors and protective factors so that students are more protected than at risk.

Times of Greatest Risk

It is especially important to support high-risk students during times of major life transitions. The need to be included and to belong is important to all of us, but for these students, during these times, it is crucial. These times include the following:

- Parents' divorcing
- Changing schools
- Moving
- A sudden illness of the student or a family member
- A stressful environment (e.g., bullying)

Role of School Nurses in Preventive Programs for High-Risk Students

- Be available to everyone. Keep your door open and the atmosphere in your office warm and inviting.
- Do not be afraid to befriend the student, families, and staff members you feel are at risk.
- Build a support system within the school (you, classroom teachers, peer advisors, guidance counselors, administrators).
- Develop a plan:
  - Identify the risk factor(s).
  - Set goals for students.
  - Provide a "safe" place for students to go. Allow them access to your office whenever the need arises without them having to state a specific illness.
  - Analyze students' day(s) and remove or relieve stressful factors (e.g., an uncompromising teacher or peer bullying).
- Evaluate students' progress as needed and revise your plans accordingly.
- Reassure students that you sincerely care about their well-being and that each of them is an important part of the school.

INTERVENTION PROGRAMS FOR THOSE ALREADY DRUG DEPENDENT

Once a student has been identified as having a drug problem, the school district's policies and procedures will dictate when the student is to be excluded, how the student is to be monitored during the recovery period, and when the student can be readmitted to school. Follow-up will also be addressed, and the school nurse will continue to be involved. This is the time when you need to be more diligent than ever. You do not want this child to be truant or to drop out of school. Treat the addicted child's absence with the same concern you demonstrate for any child with a chronic illness. You can make the difference in this student's recovery.

Role of School Nurses in Intervention Programs for Those Already Drug Dependent

- Encourage the student to return to school as soon as possible.
- Welcome the student back and set aside time in your day to see the student, and help him or her to readjust and catch up on missed schoolwork.
- Keep in touch with the home, family physician, and any outside agency involved.
- Remain discrete. Know where to document drug-related information and do not violate your district's policy on confidentiality.

═══════════════════════════*FAST FACTS in a NUTSHELL*

Do not attempt to counsel a student on your own. This is not your role. Work with the school's team of professionals and implement the school policies and procedures.

Clinical Snapshot

Helen reports her concerns to the guidance and drug counselors at school. Together they meet with David's parents to explain what they suspect.

Parents will frequently confide in you seeking your approval and support. Maintain professional boundaries, listen, and encourage them to seek appropriate services, in or out of school.

WHY SCHOOLS HAVE SO MUCH RESPONSIBILITY IN THIS AREA

The reader might now be thinking, Why does the school (and I, myself, in particular) have such a great responsibility? What about the parents, family members, other teachers, the community, and religious institutions? Consider the following facts:

- Children must attend school for approximately 5 hours a day, which is far more time than many of them spend with their parents. Students are a captive audience for us.
- As with most health topics, drug education *should* be taught at home. The sad fact is, however, that it is not. We must pick up that slack.
- Parents are sometimes not the best role models. *You are.* You made that decision when you chose a health profession, and you renewed that commitment when you started your school nursing career.

As far as the health needs of your students are concerned, as always, you know what is best.

15

School Violence

The responsibility that schools have in educating today's children is enormous. Helping them reach the point of self-actualization is an exciting challenge. It is important to remember that no matter how well a curriculum is written, how skillfully a teacher instructs, or how elaborate a school facility is, children will not grow academically and emotionally unless their basic needs for safety and belonging have first been met.

In this chapter, you will learn:

1. Maslow's theory on the hierarchy of needs
2. The scope of violence in today's schools and society in general
3. Factors that can increase the risk of violent behavior
4. Levels of violent behavior
5. Possible contributing factors to violent acts
6. Strategies that can be implemented in schools to decrease violence

MASLOW'S HIERARCHY OF NEEDS

In a 1943 manuscript entitled "A Theory of Human Motivation," psychologist Abraham Maslow speculated that there is a hierarchy of human needs. Dr. Maslow represented these needs in the form of a pyramid that is still referenced today for its significant influence on education (see Figure 15.1).

The basic elements of this theory are as follows:

- As with all animals, humans' basic needs are instinctive.
- People start with weak dispositions that are developed as they grow.
- If the environment is right, a person grows straight, beautiful, and to his or full potential.
- If the environment is not right, a person cannot progress to a higher level.
- A person does not even feel the need for the next level until the previous need has been satisfied.

Basic physiological needs such as water, food, oxygen, and constant body temperature form the foundation or bottom of the pyramid. Just above that are safety needs, including a secure environment and freedom from physical and mental harm. Once a person's physiological needs are met and he or she feels safe, the person seeks to receive and give love and affection, and to find a place where he or she belongs. Only when a person's biological, safety, and sense-of-belonging needs are addressed will that person develop self-esteem.

Lastly, when all the foregoing needs are fully satisfied, a person will achieve self-actualization. This is a state in which the person is comfortable with himself or herself in the current environment and is free to do what he or she was "born to do."

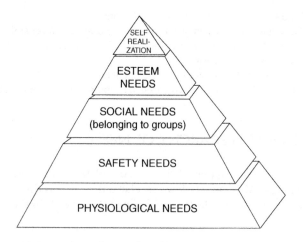

Figure 15.1 Maslow's hierarchy of basic human needs.

According to statistical data from the National Crime Victimization Survey in 2007, 4 out of every 1,000 students had experienced a serious violent crime. In data released by the National Center for Education Statistics (2009), 10% of boys and 5% of girls had been threatened or injured with a weapon while at school.

Bullying remains the most frequently reported disciplinary problem in schools. According to information provided in "Indicators of School Crime and Safety: 2009" (National Center for Education Statistics, 2009), 42.9% of sixth-grade boys and 14.4% of sixth-grade girls were being bullied and physically injured. Because bullying is so commonplace and ranges in severity, its impact is very often overlooked.

Healthy People 2020 Objectives

Injury and Violence Prevention, 35

Reduce the percentage of students in grades 9 through 12 who reported that they were bullied on school property in the previous 12 months from 17.97% in 2009 to 17.9%.

FAST FACTS in a NUTSHELL

Violence is defined as the intentional use of physical force or power against another person, group, or community with the behavior likely to cause physical or psychological harm (CDC, 2014b). A violent act always has a victim, who can be another student, a teacher, or a staff member. A student might be a victim, a perpetrator, or both.

The sad truth is that as long as violence occurs in our society, it will also occur in our schools. Schools simply mirror what is going on in the community or larger world.

Clinical Snapshot

Joseph is a student with severe behavioral issues. He is one of a number of 10th graders who belong to a gang allegedly responsible for numerous acts of violence in the community. School nurse Theresa is aware that he has served time in a juvenile detention center and is now returning to school on probation. Theresa must be part of the team planning his reentrance back to the school community. Careful monitoring is essential here.

VIOLENCE IN SOCIETY

There are four general areas where violent behavior is manifested: in the home, on the street, in gangs, and anywhere that emotional or sexual abuse occurs. A child might live in a home that is violent or one in which he or she is exposed to degenerate acts in the media. The child might witness violent behavior between or among adults or children of any age. Violent acts could include an intentional vendetta, an accidental injury or death, or an injury or death that is self-inflicted.

Today's children live in a complex society. Family, community, friends, and teachers all have varying degrees of influence on them. No matter how well-connected school nurses are with students, much that occurs in their lives is invisible to us. We may suspect problems, but unless children are willing to break their self-imposed walls of silence and speak honestly, much of the turmoil will remain unknown to us.

As long as people gather together in places such as schools, there will be both tender gestures of friendship and terrible acts of cruelty. We are all capable of both kindness and violence. Often, an act of cruelty occurs as part of a group experience, the outgrowth of a child's desperate need to be part of a social group, which is a natural drive in the development of the child.

Sadly, to fit in and be accepted, children often feel compelled to perform acts that they would not normally consider, or to exclude and victimize others. This can, and often does, lead to acts of a violent nature.

FACTORS INCREASING THE RISK OF A STUDENT BEING VIOLENT

Following any tragically violent incident perpetrated by a student, the previously overlooked warning signs become clear. Usually, the violence was generated in one of three areas of the student's life: home, school, or personal behavior. The following factors were identified by Davidson in his book *School Conflict* (2003, pp. 34–35):

Home-Life Factors

- Being physically abused
- Witnessing domestic violence

- Having a parent abuse alcohol or drugs
- Having a parent with mental illness
- Experiencing extreme family stress
- Having to move frequently
- Living in poverty

School Factors

- Being bullied
- Feeling humiliated or disrespected
- Feeling isolated or excluded
- Earning poor grades
- Lacking interest in school or community activities
- Feeling disconnected from adults

Personal-Behavior Factors

- Displaying an inability to control anger
- Abusing alcohol or drugs
- Carrying a weapon
- Belonging to a gang
- Deriving pleasure from hurting people or animals
- Participating in vandalism
- Lacking problem-solving and communication skills
- Experiencing a decline in respect for life and authority
- Having low self-esteem
- Being mentally ill or mentally disabled

LEVELS OF VIOLENT BEHAVIOR

Violent behavior can be best understood as occurring at different levels across a spectrum, which includes teasing and bullying.

Teasing

Teasing may involve verbal or nonverbal behaviors. Usually, it is considered to be a playful and harmless means of interpersonal interaction. However, everyone responds differently to teasing, and reactions are hard to predit. Teasing can lead to bullying.

Bullying

Bullying is a behavior that can be verbal or nonverbal, and it can progress to physical actions. Bullying involves intended harm, repetition, and one person or group overpowering another. The actions and results of bullying can be mild, moderate, or severe. Shoving, put-downs, name-calling, and excluding a person from the group are examples of bullying at a mild level. These behaviors can escalate quickly to intimidation, damaging property, making threats, spreading rumors, punching, or tripping.

Severe bullying involves fighting, using—or threatening to use—weapons, demanding money, extortion, stealing, destroying property, assault, prejudice, locker theft, gang activity, and bomb use. Obviously, homicide and causing suicide are the ultimate acts of violence.

FAST FACTS in a NUTSHELL

Children who are bullied may experience a variety of symptoms, including insomnia, depression, anxiety disorders, headaches, and stomachaches. These children are frequently absent from school, are tardy, skip classes, and exhibit school phobias. Often, they drop out of school altogether rather than having to constantly face the perpetrator(s).

Clinical Snapshot

Theresa begins to look into Joseph's past school experiences and contacts his elementary school nurse. She learns that Joseph was frequently absent and has a family with a history of violent behavior. Joseph was often seen in the health office and did not socialize with the other children. The elementary nurse also indicated that Joseph was teased and bullied by other children.

Theresa could strive to better understand Joseph's current behavior and work to help Joseph find a place in school where he could be comfortable.

POSSIBLE CONTRIBUTING FACTORS TO VIOLENT BEHAVIOR

No one knows for certain exactly what causes students to act violently. Some possible reasons include:

- Lack of nurturing
- Schools that permit corporal punishment
- Large-scale political protests
- Increased use of drugs
- Violent, unstable family life
- Increased number of divorces and single-parent homes
- Transient population
- Graphic movies, song lyrics, and video games
- Easier access to guns and other weapons
- Internet communication

FAST FACTS in a NUTSHELL

Violence and bullying have received increasing attention due to a number of nationally publicized incidents. Be mindful that serious problems often begin with teasing and can escalate quickly.

Clinical Snapshot

Joseph's problems should have been addressed earlier. Unfortunately, no adult was alert or cared enough to help him. Seldom will a child complain about being teased. The adult in authority must be alert for evidence that it is occurring. Encourage teachers to establish strict, classroom rules and reasonable consequences for unwanted teasing. Question those you believe are being bullied and seek immediate disciple for those doing the bullying.

STRATEGIES TO KEEP SCHOOLS SAFE

There are three basic approaches to preventing school violence.

1. *Educational and curriculum-based initiatives (primary prevention):* These approaches include character-building education programs, conflict-resolution lessons, development of a student code of school conduct, and gang-prevention discussions. When used appropriately, primary preventive strategies are most effective.

2. *School management initiatives (secondary prevention)*: School management includes means and methods of discipline and punishment for threats—and actual acts—of violence. All acts of violence must be reported to the appropriate authorities. Those in authority must adopt a zero-tolerance stance. This means that all incidents are dealt with as severely as school policy and state and federal laws permit.

3. *School environment modification (tertiary prevention)*: This includes the installation of video surveillance cameras, closed-circuit televisions, security locks, metal detectors, scanners, identification cards, security guards, and school uniforms.

Violence frequently centers around one of the following issues:

- Jealousy over a boyfriend or girlfriend
- Peer pressure
- Revenge
- Confrontation
- Drug influence
- Racial or ethnic prejudice
- Gang territorial issues

ROLE OF SCHOOL NURSES IN PREVENTING AND DEALING WITH SCHOOL VIOLENCE

- Get to know your students. Gain their trust.
- Promote a school climate where students are listened to and respected.
- Insist on zero tolerance for *all* acts of violence. If bullying and other acts of violence are not addressed, you are condoning them.
- Check on students' social behaviors to and from school, on the school bus, and during after-school activities.
- Encourage students to talk to you. Be alert for threats of violent behavior. Listen for any vague threats.
- Be alert for danger signs in a student who:
  - Does not fit in socially
  - Shows no interest in activities, self, or peers
  - Suddenly gets poor grades
  - Is depressed
  - Appears to be obsessed with violence and death
  - Carries weapons to school
  - Has poor anger-management skills

  - Writes about or makes drawings expressing despair
  - Is cruel to animals
  - Has frequent mood swings
- Use teachable moments to communicate with students.
- Maintain your office as a safe refuge for all. Allow students to "cool off" or escape for a few minutes when they need to.
- Initiate antiviolence clubs.
- Encourage peer-mediation procedures.
- Be part of school and community task forces that deal with violence.
- Prioritize victims and their needs. Question whether perpetrators are also victims.
- Arrange staff education about preventing violence *before* there is a tragic incident.
- Help every student connect or fit in someplace and with someone.
- Investigate every student's frequent absences and repeated visits to your office.
- Insist that incidences of violence be reported to the proper authorities.
- Recognize when information must be shared to protect a student.
- Suggest periodic patrolling of the areas that are normally not well supervised: the lunchroom, halls, bathroom, playground, and so on.
- Reward acts of kindness.

16

Child Abuse

At one time, people might have thought that there was no such thing as child abuse. Prior to compulsory school attendance, many were oblivious to what was going on in homes across the country. However, as large numbers of students gathered in schools comparisons among children became inevitable. School personnel were able to clearly identify the students who were happy and thriving in their home and school environments, and those who were not. Schools today now play an important role in early detection of child abuse.

The sooner child abuse is recognized and reported, and help is provided to the family, the greater is the chance that the child will heal and not perpetuate the cycle.

In this chapter, you will learn:

1. Definitions of institutional and noninstitutional child abuse
2. Major aspects of the Child Abuse Prevention and Treatment Act
3. Types of child abuse and neglect, along with warning signs, risk factors, and prevention strategies
4. Basic referral processes and the school's responsibility in documenting and reporting suspicions of child abuse and neglect

DEFINITIONS OF CHILD ABUSE

Broadly defined, *child abuse* is an omission of nurturing. Abuse includes much more than physical harm. In the past, when people thought of child abuse, many immediately imagined a child with visible bruises and broken bones. As distressing as this image is, there are less obvious, but equally damaging, types of child abuse that are far more common. These leave deep, long-lasting scars that have a ripple effect on families from past to present generations and generations yet to come.

One problem regarding child abuse today, as in earlier days, is how to distinguish abuse from overzealous parenting or teaching that intentionally or accidentally causes injury. There is still no consensus as to exactly what constitutes effective parental and school discipline and what constitutes abuse.

INSTITUTIONAL AND NONINSTITUTIONAL CHILD ABUSE

Child abuse can occur anywhere and anytime. The abuser can be a stranger, teacher, trusted friend, family member, priest, rabbi, scout leader, caretaker, school employee, or health care provider.

Institutional abuse occurs when an act of abuse takes place in a school or any formal institutional facility. The perpetrator might be a staff member, teacher, principal, older student, or custodian. Each school district has in place policies and procedures to deal with allegations of abuse by staff members and other employees.

Noninstitutional abuse occurs in homes. The perpetrator is usually a parent, relative, or someone else whom a parent has entrusted to watch the child.

FAST FACTS in a NUTSHELL

Each state has specific laws addressing child abuse. All states require that knowledge of alleged offenses or suspected incidences of child abuse be reported by school personnel, regardless of where these alleged offenses or incidences occurred or by whom they were committed.

Clinical Snapshot

Eight-year-old Jorge arrives in school with a lacerated lip and profuse nosebleed. Jorge states his mother hit him because he would not finish breakfast. Jorge's mom is a close friend of School Nurse Margaret and she is certain he is lying. She calls home to have mom come and take him to be evaluated for suturing. When Jorge's mother arrives at school, she explains that he fell. Margaret accepts her word and does not refer the incident to child protective services.

The following week Jorge arrives at school with several teeth missing. He again states that his mother hit him. Margaret now makes the referral, angry with herself that she allowed a friendship to interfere with following proper procedure, heartsick that she permitted a child to go home to an unsafe environment, and fearful that she has left herself liable for failing to report suspicion of child abuse.

Healthy People 2020 Objectives

Injury and Violence Prevention, 38

Reduce nonfatal maltreatment from 9.4% per 1,000 children under age 18 years in 2008 to 8.5%.

CHILD ABUSE PREVENTION AND TREATMENT ACT

The Child Abuse Prevention and Treatment Act (CAPTA) was passed in 1974 and reauthorized in 2010. It covers all persons under 18 years of age. CAPTA defines *child abuse* as:

. . . at a minimum, any recent act or failure to act on the part of a parent or caretaker which results in death, serious physical or emotional harm, sexual abuse or exploitation, or an act or failure to act which presents an imminent risk of serious harm.

CAPTA provides federal money to all states to help implement programs that identify, treat, and prevent child abuse. To be granted this money, states must do the following:

- Indicate who are considered the reporters
- Offer a clear definition of *maltreatment*
- Identify the agreed-upon procedure for reporting suspected abuse and neglect
- Indicate the agency that will receive and investigate the reports
- Provide immunity from prosecution for good-faith reporters

- Provide penalties for failure to report, as well as for the issuing of false reports (misdemeanors punishable by fines or imprisonment, or both)
- Include additional provisions that nullify certain communication rights
- Add additional provisions unique to the state

CATEGORIES OF CHILD ABUSE

There are four general classifications of child abuse: physical abuse, sexual abuse, emotional abuse, and neglect. Any of these may occur separately, but they more often occur in combination. All have devastating emotional impacts on children and severely limit their ability to learn. The descriptions and lists of indicators that follow were adapted from the National Children's Advocacy Center (2010), the Child Welfare Information Gateway (2013), and the Centers for Disease Control and Prevention (CDC, 2013b).

Physical Abuse

Physical abuse is reported most frequently because bruises and broken bones are visibly obvious and immediately raise suspicions. Such abuse involves physical harm or injury, which may be intentional or a result of severe discipline. Family background and cultural traditions play a role in physical abuse patterns. Some parents insist that it is their right and responsibility to use force to teach their children right from wrong. Physical abuse includes punching, beating, shaking, or hitting a victim with the hand or an object. Such victims learn to live in fear.

Physical indicators: Unexplained bruises, abrasions, fractures, lacerations, or welts
Behavioral indicators: Anxiety about going home, wariness of adults, extreme withdrawal or aggressiveness, fear of the perpetrator, frequent reports of injuries by parents, the wearing of seasonally inappropriate clothing to cover arms or legs, and self-destructive actions

Sexual Abuse

Sexual abuse includes actions by a perpetrator such as inappropriate touching of the breasts or genitals, actual penetration, incest, rape, sodomy, indecent exposure, and exploitation through prostitution or the production of pornographic materials. Sexual abuse does not necessarily involve bodily contact. A child's exposure to sexual situations or materials is also considered to be abuse.

Physical indicators: Urinary tract infections; difficulty walking or sitting; torn, stained, or bloody underclothing; pain or itching in the genital area; bruises or bleeding in the external genitalia; venereal disease; and pregnancy

Behavioral indicators: Extreme modesty; withdrawn behavior; fantasized or infantile behavior; bizarre, sophisticated, or unusual sexual behavior; poor peer relationships; delinquent or runaway behavior; reports of sexual assault; suicide attempts; and extreme weight change

FAST FACTS in a NUTSHELL

Sexual abuse is especially frightening because it frequently remains hidden and creates feelings of guilt and shame in the victim. Usually, the offender is someone the child knows and trusts. The child often feels responsible and may experience sexual problems as he or she gets older.

Clinical Snapshot

Jorge's mom has a live-in boyfriend whom Jorge clearly fears. You notice that Jorge frequently stops in to see you after school to delay going home. Margaret needs to ask Jorge the hard questions. Is he afraid to go home? Why does he dislike his mother's boyfriend? Has his mother's boyfriend ever tried to touch him inappropriately?

Emotional Abuse

Emotional abuse can severely damage a child's self-esteem and social development. Such abuse is usually repetitive and includes verbal insults or severe punishment. The scars are lifelong and can lead to psychiatric issues. The impact of emotional abuse can be even greater than sexual or physical abuse. Examples of emotional abuse include constant belittling, humiliating, name-calling, threatening, bullying, ignoring, and rejecting a child as punishment; limited physical contact (e.g., lack of hugging, kissing, and affection); and exposing a child to violence or abuse by others.

Physical indicators: Habit disorders such as sucking, biting, or rocking; conduct disorders such as antisocial or destructive behavior; and neurotic traits, including sleep disorders, speech disorders, and inhibition of play

Behavioral indicators: Behavior extremes, overly adaptive behavior, and attempted suicide

Neglect

Child neglect is the failure to provide for a child's basic needs. Neglect is not often reported or apparent to the casual observer. Children have a remarkable way of adapting, and they may blame themselves for a lack of nurturing from their parents. Many more children experience neglect than are either physically or sexually abused.

Areas of Child Neglect

- *Physical neglect:* Failure to provide adequate food, clothing, shelter, or supervision
- *Medical neglect:* Failure to provide needed medical care
- *Educational neglect:* Failure to provide education or to tend to the special needs of a child
- *Emotional neglect:* Failure to tend to a child's emotional needs or to provide psychological care, or permitting a child to use alcohol or drugs

Neglect is the most common form of child abuse. Many teachers will simply choose to ignore it rather than jeopardize their relationship with the parent. You will be able to help in this area better than anyone else in the school.

Physical indicators: Hunger, poor hygiene, inappropriate clothing, lack of supervision, fatigue, unattended physical problems or medical needs, and abandonment

Behavioral indicators: Begging, stealing food or other items, reluctance to leave school, falling asleep in class, substance abuse, delinquency, dropping out of school, and no known caregiver

As professional caregivers we find it difficult to fathom that some children are abused and neglected by their parents. Many parents are also tolerant of abuse that occurs in schools. Some parents even encourage teachers to use physical punishment, completely trusting the staff and believing that such punishment will benefit their children.

What is especially upsetting is that society as a whole must acknowledge being a part of creating and maintaining an atmosphere that may lead to child abuse. Poverty, transient lifestyles, single parenting, overexposure to violence in the media, and inadequate child protective service agencies all contribute to an environment that increases the likelihood of neglect and abuse. The horror of child abuse, therefore, is not a simple issue that exists only between the victim and the perpetrator. We must look at the bigger picture and the role that we play in it.

RISK FACTORS FOR CHILD ABUSE

As recognized by Saisan and Segal (2010), certain conditions or situations place students at risk for abuse. They include the following:

Poverty: All too often, adequate services are not available to poor families. When a parent is unemployed or ill, the family may have inadequate food, clothing, and shelter. Poor people tend to move frequently, causing further unease. In addition, most illegal immigrants are afraid to report their needs lest they be deported.

Violence in the home: It is terrifying for a child to witness violence among family members. Children suffer tremendous emotional damage when they are subjected to violence in the home.

Parental history of abuse: If either parent has been abused, it is likely that he or she will perpetuate the abuse cycle.

Lack of parenting skills: Parents who are very young, mentally unstable, or have never had good role models often do not know how to nurture their children properly.

Mental illness: If they are not diagnosed and treated, parents with mental illness may direct their anger and frustrations toward their children.

Transient lifestyle: Parents who often move from place to place may not live near other family members, and therefore they have little or no support.

Substance abuse: Parents who are substance abusers are often child abusers as well. Their judgment is poor and inconsistent.

PREVENTION STRATEGIES

As with many other issues, prevention is the key, and education is the only way to achieve it.

Education of Staff

This can be done through yearly educational programs so that teachers and staff can recognize the signs of child abuse and neglect, and understand their role in the process of prevention, detection, and referral.

Education for Students

Children need to be empowered with information to protect themselves. The best way to accomplish this is to offer a comprehensive school health curriculum focusing on prevention strategies for children.

Education for Parents

In some cases, parents need outside resources to cope with parenting in appropriate ways. Counseling services and educational programs are available, and the school nurse can facilitate parental access. Parents need to know that it is the law that all *suspected* cases of child abuse and neglect must be reported.

FAST FACTS in a NUTSHELL

After Margaret makes the call to Children's Protective Services, she informs the principal of her actions. Within five minutes the classroom teacher is in her office complaining that she had not been informed.

Be clear as to which administrator you will share information with. Remain discrete and keep *only* that person informed. You tend to the needs of the child; let administrators take care of staff and each other. Check your state's policy. If you believe you will be penalized for reporting a suspicion of abuse, you may not have to inform any school administrator.

🔘 Clinical Snapshot

Jorge also shares with you that his 19-year-old, cousin is always trying to get him alone to kiss and touch his *private parts*. Margaret makes the referral and inform the principal that a representative from child protective services is coming to the school. The guidance counselor, secretaries, and custodial staff want to know what is going on. Out of respect for the child and family members, Margaret does not share this information. Instead, she refers them to the principal.

═══════════════════════════════*FAST FACTS in a NUTSHELL*

Calling a child protective services agency is a difficult thing to do. Many people just do not want to get involved. Any nurse with this attitude should find a specialty other than that of school nursing. Protecting children is part of a school nurse's job, and the nurse "got involved" on the day that he or she chose school nursing.

🔘 Clinical Snapshot

Margaret checks her mailbox just before leaving school for the weekend. She finds a note from a third-grade teacher informing her of an alleged incident of noninstitutional sexual abuse involving one of her students that was reported to the teacher that morning. The teacher asks her to *look into it*. The teacher, student, and building administrator have already left for the weekend. Margaret is furious with the teacher but returns to your office and makes the referral call, knowing that she has acted in the best interest of that child. Margaret notifies the teacher and principal that she expects to meet with them to discuss their professional responsibilities.

BASIC REFERRAL PROCESS

Most states have regulations requiring the "first person contact" to make a referral. This means that whoever speaks with a child *first* about abuse or neglect, or whoever has a strong suspicion that abuse is occurring, must report it to the proper agency themselves. You can assist reporters of abuse or neglect by providing the appropriate phone numbers and any history of the child that you are aware of, but the responsibility to call is *theirs*.

The steps in this process are as follows:

1. You or another adult has *reasonable cause* to believe that a child is being abused or neglected. If a child has a visible bruise, and states, "My father hit me," then it is clear that a referral is necessary. Many cases are not as obvious. A child might be afraid to admit that a parent hurt him or her lest this anger the parent or cause the child to be removed from the home.

2. In good faith, the child protective services agency is notified. If you are uncertain whether the child was hit by the parent, you can explain that to the caseworker, who will investigate.

3. Provide the agency with the necessary information: the child's name, address, the names of any siblings, the parents' names, phone numbers, workplaces, and so on.

4. Make the call early in the day if possible. Often, an investigator will need to come to the school to speak with the child.

5. Insist on seeing identification from anyone asking to speak with the child in school and remain present to support the child.

6. Document according to district policy.

7. Follow up on all referrals.

ROLE OF SCHOOL NURSES IN CHILD ABUSE

Preventive Strategies

- Be alert to the risk factors in a child's life.
- Recognize the early signs, symptoms, and behavioral indicators of child neglect and abuse.
- Know your district's policy on reporting child abuse.
- Arrange staff educational programs. Teach the signs and symptoms of child abuse to the entire staff: teachers, lunch aides, classroom aides, bus drivers, after-school personnel, coaches, and so on.
- Caution staff members not to place themselves in positions where they are alone with students and can be accused of child abuse.
- Develop a zero-tolerance approach for child abuse and neglect.

- Make certain that information about the individual's right to privacy and protection of his or her own body is provided to students via the health education curriculum.
- Inform all parents and staff, in writing and publicly at meetings, that the first person contact *by law* is to report all incidents of suspected child abuse.
- Accept that this part of your job is ugly, but it must be done.

Detection and Reporting Strategies

- Be available to listen and ready to ask the difficult questions.
- When speaking with a child, use objective, not leading, questioning techniques: "Tell me about that bruise" as opposed to "Who hit you?"
- Seek only enough information to formulate a suspicion. Do not interrogate.
- Immediately report all suspicions of child abuse to the proper authorities. Do not examine the child unless there is a specific complaint of injury.
- Insist on counseling for child and parent.
- Work with police and community agencies.
- Insist that staff report suspicions to the proper authorities.
- Document objectively according to your district and state regulations so there is no room for multiple interpretations.
- Do not allow a child to go home to an unsafe environment. Do not transport a child in your car. Consult local law enforcement agency for assistance.
- *Do not call the parents* unless directed to do so by the protective agency.
- If the investigator from the child protective services agency feels that an investigation is not warranted and you strongly disagree, speak with another investigator or supervisor. Keep asking for an investigation until someone listens.
- Keep notes on the referral in a confidential file. It may be necessary to retrieve this information years later.

17

Cultural Diversity

If you have ever read historical memoirs of famous generals, you can appreciate how carefully war plans are made. Prior to any battle, extensive research goes into understanding the enemy's religion, ethnicity, and all other aspects of the culture. A plan is formulated, the ground force is established, war is waged, and the opponent is defeated. Only by thinking like the enemy can the war be won. As generals leading the struggle for the success of all our children, we have the responsibility to mobilize all school resources to help prepare and protect children from the enemies they will face.

Immigrant families arrive in this country with enemies. These enemies are in the form of risk factors such as poverty, social isolation, language barriers, different lifestyles, and few, if any, extended family members to support them. All of these can impede a child's ability to learn. They can win over the child and prevent him or her from thriving unless our society can help to overcome their virulent influence.

School is where these different students meet and ideally, learn, with—and about—each other. It is essential that school personnel respect diversity and celebrate the richness that cultural, racial, and ethnic diversity brings to the school.

In this chapter, you will learn:

1. Definitions of culture and diversity
2. The challenges of cultural diversity in American schools
3. Cultural sensitivity and competency for diverse school populations
4. Steps to foster academic achievement for students with diverse backgrounds

CULTURE

Culture cannot be defined in just a few words; numerous theories and models have been developed over the years. However, to summarize, culture is:

- Learned behavior that guides thinking, decisions, and activities in a predictable way
- Shared patterns of beliefs, values, and actions
- An inclusive term that covers ethnicity, race, national origin, and religion
- Various traditions that are shared and passed along
- A guide for dealing with other people
- A means to pass values from one generation to another
- A group of students who share the same interests within the class structure; artists, athletes, cheerleaders, and musicians, for example, might be considered separate cultural groups

As our country continues to become ever more culturally and ethnically diverse, so do our schools. Therefore, within any large school, there are many different ethnic groups, various languages spoken, and unique cultural attitudes toward education. As the blending of people of different ethnic and racial backgrounds increases in the years to come, it is projected that today's minority populations will become the majority.

At issue today is how to meet the educational needs of so many culturally diverse children. Extremely poor minority children might be at risk for learning disabilities as a result of deprivation or emotional trauma. However, the vast majority of them are perfectly capable of learning as other children do. It is not the ability that they lack, it is the rich experiences that so many other children are afforded in this country today.

Lack of understanding on the part of educators, inadequate communication, and inaccurate evaluations may lead us to label minority students unfairly. School professionals frequently fail to understand and respect different cultural traditions and lack the wisdom to work effectively with various ethnic groups.

Healthy People 2020 Objectives

Educational and Community-Based Programs, 14.2

Increase the inclusion of cultural diversity content in undergraduate nursing programs from 98% in 2009 to 100%.

Diversity is a good thing, provided we develop understanding and respect for one another's differences. The goals are to recognize and appreciate the differences, establish helping relationships, see to it that every child succeeds academically, and emotionally finds a comfortable place in the school environment.

Diversity exists in almost every classroom in any school in this country. There are students from different states, countries, and cultures. *Diversity* simply means that differences exist. Differences can include the following:

- Race
- Language
- Ethnicity
- Sexual orientation
- Level or type of education
- Nationality
- Hobbies or interests
- Religion
- Socioeconomic status
- Thinking processes

═══════════════ *FAST FACTS in a NUTSHELL*

As the community is diverse, so will be your schools. And just as the community climate of acceptance influences the school, so, too, does the school influence the community.

🌀 Clinical Snapshot

Sanjay is a fourth-grade student who recently immigrated from India. School nurse Susan notices that he refuses to eat lunch in school. He is qualified for a free lunch program but brings a brown bag that is never opened. After questioning Sanjay, Susan finds that he dislikes the cafeteria offerings and is afraid others will laugh at what he brings from home. Susan arranges for him to eat at the same table as another Indian student who is familiar with his food choices and where he can gradually grow more accustomed to the American diet.

Demographics

According to Klauke (1989), an estimated half of the children in the nation's schools are of African, Asian, or Hispanic origin. In some states, such as Hawaii, New Mexico, and California, the percentages are even higher. Experts predict that most future immigrants will arrive from Asia and Latin America, and they will continue to settle in metropolitan areas such as New York, Los Angeles, and Chicago. These cities and many others include tremendous diversity in cultures, economic status, educational levels, and family values. This is where the challenge begins.

BENEFITS OF CULTURAL DIVERSITY IN SCHOOLS

In a proper school setting, with capable, enthusiastic teachers, there are many benefits to having diverse student populations, as described in the following list.

- *Students are more accepting of differences:* When students learn in a diverse environment at an early age, they become more tolerant and accepting.
- *Students experience freedom from prejudices:* By working together, side by side every day, children learn not to form prejudices or feelings of superiority.
- *Education is promoted and enhanced:* Children learn from each other. They learn cultural tolerance and acceptance as well as academics.
- *Students experience minimum adjustment issues:* When they have been exposed to different cultures at an early age, children are prepared for life beyond school and in an ever more blended world.
- *Patriotism is promoted for all:* When students have the opportunity to learn about other cultures, ideally, they compare and appreciate the learning opportunities that they have been allowed to have in this country (Borkar, 2010).

CHALLENGES OF CULTURAL DIVERSITY IN SCHOOLS

Integrating diverse cultures is a challenge. To be successful, some issues must be addressed within a school environment, such as those described in the following list:

- *Teachers' attitudes:* Teachers and other staff members must be willing to extend themselves to address the unique needs of each student.
- *Administrative support:* Teachers need support to help communicate with students and parents. Any necessary additional services (interpreters, counselors, etc.) should be provided to them.
- *Proper screening and evaluation procedures:* The multidisciplinary team must be sensitive to every family's needs and flexible in their approach.
- *Staff training:* Education must be provided to all staff members who have contact with culturally diverse students.
- *School and community environment:* Prejudice leading to bullying that escalates to violence is a very real threat to minority students. Members of the school and community must be aware of this and seek to minimize or eliminate this type of threat.
- *Financial burden for school districts:* Without question, the multiple needs of minority students place a financial burden on school districts. Preventive initiatives such as preschool programs and counseling are less costly than intervention programs. These must be offered at any cost by the school district, or the state or federal government.

CULTURAL SENSITIVITY AND COMPETENCY

Cultural sensitivity can be defined as having an open attitude toward a culture or ethnic background different from one's own. It is a prerequisite to cultural competence. Cultural competency is the ability to interact effectively with people of other cultures, which grows out of an understanding of and respect for the culture, beliefs, and practices of other people. Because cultural competency is a process, it is enhanced and increases as we grow and learn in our profession.

Steps Toward Cultural Competency

- Self-reflection
- Attaining information about different cultures
- Developing respect and understanding
- Remaining nonjudgmental
- Revising methods of dealing with students as needed

FAST FACTS in a NUTSHELL

Some school personnel never achieve cultural competence. Know who these individuals are and continue to advocate for your students.

Clinical Snapshot

Mrs. G., a third grade teacher who has taught for decades, repeatedly complains about the increasing number of non-English speaking students. Susan feels sorry for the students placed in her class.

Teachers can become frustrated when trying to communicate with non–English-speaking students and parents. Recommend that non–English-speaking students be placed with teachers who are more understanding. Ensure that interpreters are available when you take a medical history or a parent–teacher conference is planned.

Barriers to Cultural Competency

- *Language:* If necessary, a school district must employ an interpreter to facilitate communication.
- *Ethnic and religious practices:* These may interfere with school policies and expectations.
- *A child's previous experiences:* A child may have witnessed violence or extreme poverty, which will likely affect his or her ability to learn. This must be addressed through counseling.

STEPS TO FOSTER ACADEMIC ACHIEVEMENT

- Keep students in school. Preventing failure is a major step in helping students avoid poverty and issues of low self-worth.
- Encourage attendance at preschool programs. These years are important in building a learning foundation and identifying children with special needs early, so that intervention can be started.
- Make sure children are evaluated fairly and without any bias.
- Work as a team with other professionals in the community and school district.

- Help students to connect with the school, staff, and other students.
- Encourage staff education.

ROLE OF SCHOOL NURSES IN DEALING WITH CULTURALLY DIVERSE STUDENTS

- Reflect on your own feelings regarding each culture of students.
- Research information on the various ethnic groups within your school.
- Work toward personally becoming culturally competent.
- Help organize staff educational programs.
- Serve on multidisciplinary teams and advocate for children from other cultures.
- Serve as a liaison between school, students, and parents.
- Help promote an atmosphere of respect, cooperation, and acceptance throughout the school.
- Provide opportunities for students and staff to celebrate cultural pride.
- Continue to offer your office and self as a refuge for all who need a safe place to visit.
- Remain cognizant of the underlying issues of great concern for immigrant children: housing, transportation, access to health care, counseling services, poverty, ethnic prejudice, and so on.

18

Disaster Planning

Every nurse knows what an emergency is. Nurses have been educated and are ready to recognize a serious threat, deal with the acute phase, help in the recovery process, and then work to prevent future similar incidents by reflecting on the why and how of the emergency.

In school nursing practice, nurses have emergency plans for certain students. We know exactly what must be done for a child who is anaphylactic, diabetic, or has a seizure disorder. There are clear protocols for children with special needs, as well as for anticipated, schoolwide emergencies such as fires and structural issues.

Nurses and many other school personnel are certified in cardiopulmonary resuscitation and automatic external defibrillator use. These skills are seldom, if ever, needed, but we are prepared in case they are.

Most school emergency situations can be planned for, responded to, and recovered from, all within the school community. A large disaster or mass casualty cannot be managed in the same way as the needs far exceed the limited resources of the school and district.

In this chapter, you will learn:

1. The definition and components of a safe school
2. How to recognize the types of disasters
3. The stages of disaster planning

A SAFE SCHOOL

In the hierarchy of needs, safety comes well before learning. We know that children can and will learn only if they feel protected. Today's schools are an integral part of the community and must be a refuge for students.

Every school district is required to have a well-written and frequently rehearsed plan that covers all the different types of mass emergencies and traumatic events.

Each local board of education is given the task of establishing policies and procedures to ensure that a sense of peace and stability remains constant in schools so that learning can take place.

FAST FACTS in a NUTSHELL

One of the first tasks you should explore when you begin work in a school district is to carefully check the safety plans for fire and mass disasters.

Clinical Snapshot

On the morning of September 11, 2001, anxious calls flooded every school in the nation. Parents sought reassurance that their children were within the safety of the school walls. Terribly shaken, many parents left their homes or workplaces to go to their children's schools so that they could see and touch their children and know they were unharmed.

The police, firefighters, and social services organizations mobilized. Hospitals near Ground Zero in New York City immediately prepared to discharge as many patients as possible to make room for anticipated casualties. Medical care facilities within the general area braced themselves for an onslaught of patients. Much of the world responded to the crisis in some manner, offering to provide any needed assistance.

Fortunately, disasters such as this are rare. However, just as we prepare for fires with fire drills and for classroom emergencies with student Emergency Care Plans, we must also be prepared for a major catastrophe.

COMPONENTS OF A SAFE SCHOOL

Addressing the issue of safety, Selekman (2006) states that schools should include:

- A focus on academic excellence
- Partnerships
- Prevention
- Intervention
- Crisis intervention
- School climate survey/assessment (pp. 206–207)

Each of the aforementioned areas has many components and requires a multidisciplinary team approach. The school nurse must participate in all such approaches and assume a prominent role.

Healthy People 2020 Objectives

Preparedness, 2

Reduce the time necessary to activate designated personnel to report for immediate duty with no advance notice from 66 minutes in 2009 to 59 minutes.

TYPES OF DISASTERS

Violence

A violent disaster involves an act of shooting, bomb planting, or suicide. Schools must recognize that bullying, depression, and self-destructive behavior are increasing. Every threat must be taken seriously and the person posing a threat referred immediately.

Terrorism and Bioterrorism

In the wake of 9/11, acts of terrorism are the foremost fear of many Americans today. One type of terrorism is bioterrorism, which is the release of small amounts of toxic biological substances that can cause tremendous harm. The following table summarizes the classification of biological agents of concern:

TABLE 18.1 Biological Agents

Risk Category	Characteristics of Agents
Category A agents (highest priority risk)*	
Botulinum toxin (Clostridium botulinum)	• Easily disseminated or transmitted from person to person
Plague (Yersinia pestis)	• High morbidity and mortality rates
Smallpox (Variola major)	• Major health impact
Tularemia (Francisella tularensis)	• Potential for public panic and social disruption
Viral hemorrhagic fevers (including Ebola, Marburg, Lassa, and Machupo)	• Require special action for public health preparedness
Category B agents (second highest priority risk)*	
Brucellosis	• Moderately easy to disseminate
Epsilon toxin of Clostridium perfringens	• Results in moderate morbidity rates and low mortality rates
Food safety threats (Salmonella, E. coli, Shigella); Melioidosis Psittacosis (Chlamydia psittaci); Q fever (Coxiella burnetii); Ricin toxin (from castor beans)	• Require specific enhancements of CDC's diagnostic capacity and enhanced disease surveillance
Staphylococcal enterotoxin B; Typhus fever (Rickettsia prowazekii); Viral encephalitis (from alphaviruses such as VEE, EEE, WEE	
Category C agents (third highest priority risk)*	
Emerging infectious diseases such as Nipah virus and hantavirus	• Availability • Ease of production and dissemination • Potential for high morbidity and mortality rates and major health impact

*According to the Centers for Disease Control and Prevention (CDC).
Source: Retrieved from cdc.gov/agent/agentlist-category.asp on March 21, 2011.

Natural and Environmental Disasters

Hurricanes, floods, earthquakes, and tornados can all be natural disasters. Although no one is to blame for such disasters, their effects are frightening and devastating, as are the effects of environmental disasters. Examples of environmental disasters include toxic exposures or spills and structural failure of a school building.

Illness

Any illness that strikes a significant percentage of the population can cause a crisis. Large numbers of people with pandemic flu or similar difficult-to-control illnesses are considered to be disasters in a community.

Also catastrophic is the sudden death of a student or staff member. Suicides are especially tragic.

DISASTER PLANNING

Factors to Consider

- The total number of people involved: students, staff, and anticipated visitors
- The number of students and staff members with special needs; note those who are wheelchair bound
- The type of disaster
- Evacuation plans
- Assembly points
- Means of communication

STAFF TRAINING

Crisis Team Members

Each local board of education must establish policies and procedures to deal with crises. The chief school administrator must put together a crisis team.

A crisis team must:

- Serve as an advisory board to the chief school administrator
- Inform school personnel of information as it develops
- Deliver services as needed

Clinical Snapshot

School nurse Sharon notes that the crisis team is planning to meet later in the afternoon. When she approaches her principal about the time and location, she is told that it is not necessary for her to attend and that there is no one to cover her office. Sharon explains the importance of her presence and suggests they try to get a substitute nurse for a couple of hours or direct the staff to send only emergencies and inform the secretary where she could be reached. Sharon feels strongly that since she is part of the solution, she should be included in the planning.

School Members

- Chief school administrator
- School psychologist
- All principals in the district
- School nurse
- Director of buildings and grounds
- Bus driver
- Guidance counselor
- Special education teacher
- School secretary
- Custodian
- Parents' organization representative
- Social worker
- Regular education teacher

Community Members

- Police department
- Fire department
- Community mental health personnel

- Emergency services personnel
- Local public officials
- Parents
- Representatives of local medical facilities

═══════════════════════════════════════ *FAST FACTS in a NUTSHELL*

Keep all disaster information and equipment in a location that is easy to access. Make sure your administrator is aware of the location and include the location in your substitute nurse's folder.

🌀 Clinical Snapshot

Sharon has an office the size of a large closet. Her *Go Kit* and other crisis necessities simply do not fit in an accessible location. It is crucial that space be allocated for these items. Perhaps a shelf can be added or a space in a nearby classroom can be designated for these essential emergency tools.

PLANNING STAGES AND SCHOOL NURSES' ROLE

There are four stages in becoming prepared for and responding to the variety of school disasters that may take place within your school environment:

1. Identify potential disasters (for your school environment)
2. Be prepared (for possible disaster types)
3. Respond (appropriately to the disaster)
4. Recover (provide recovery support, as needed)

A detailed description of these stages follows.

Identify Potential Disasters

This is primary prevention when it is most important. There is little anyone can do to avert terrorism, natural disasters, or even many environmental issues. However, violence can and should be addressed more effectively in the schools.

Role of School Nurses in Identifying Potential Disasters

- Help create a school climate that fosters an atmosphere of respect between adults and students.
- Consider offering schoolwide safety and character-education programs.
- Insist on a no-bullying policy and see that it is enforced.
- Watch the loners. Every student should fit in with someone.
- Be alert for threats.
- Find students who will inform you of classmates who make threats and are willing to break the students' code of silence.
- Insist on written physician clearance for any student returning to school after a period of depression or suicide attempt, stating that the student is not a danger to self or others.

Be Prepared

In preparation for a disaster, it is essential that consideration be given to general disaster principles and specific plans for individual schools. Each school has a different location, types and ages of students, and individual needs that will influence emergency planning.

The School Emergency Plan

The school emergency plan should be reviewed annually and updated as needed. Drills should be practiced at least yearly, meet the unique needs of the individual school, and delegate specific activities for each member of the crisis team. In addition, the school emergency plan should include the following:

- An outline of a predetermined response plan
- Provisions for trained people with knowledge and skills to act as emergency responders
- Provisions to minimize the risk of serious injury, death, or property damage
- Provisions for first aid and counseling for staff, students, parents, and community members during and after the crisis
- Provisions for accurate, up-to-date information to be given to parents, the community, and the media
- Guidelines for how to evaluate the response and revise the plan
- A goal to return the school to its normal level of function as soon as possible
- Development of a postemergency plan for the aftermath of any disaster

Types of School Disaster Drills

- Evacuation: The students must exit the building in a quick, orderly fashion, as for a threat of a fire.
- Lockdown: A lockdown is necessary when a perpetrator is believed to be present in the building or on the school grounds. Students are directed to stand clear of doors and windows, and rooms are locked.
- Drop and cover: Students are directed to take shelter under desks or against walls, with their bodies covered as much as possible. This is recommended during a natural disaster such as a hurricane or tornado.

Role of School Nurses in Preparing for a Disaster

- Ask to review the school emergency plan.
- Be part of the crisis management team.
- Assemble a *School Nurse's Go Kit*.

School Nurse's Go Kit Components

Documents:

Crisis management plan	School blueprints
Emergency cards	Individualized and emergency plans
Teacher and student class lists	Absentee list for the day
Alert list	Standing orders
Medication list for students and staff	Emergency evacuation plans
Class pictures or yearbook	Important phone numbers

Supplies:

Students' personal medications	Spill kit
Gloves, gowns	Bandages, splints, ice packs
Biohazard bags and masks	Flashlight
Communication devices	Blood pressure machine, stethoscope
Master keys for building	Hand sanitizer
Pens, paper, markers	Name tags

Respond

Once the traumatic event has occurred, intervention takes place. Ideally, plans are in place, procedures have been rehearsed, and the team is ready and available to protect the students.

ROLE OF SCHOOL NURSES IN RESPONDING TO A DISASTER

- Organize the first-aid treatment for the injured.
- Triage.
- Counsel students as needed while remaining calm.
- Make sure that those with special needs are tended to.
- Keep your *Go Kit* with you.

Recovery

After the crisis situation has passed, the school community enters the recovery phase. This is a critical time for all, and the school nurse's calm effectiveness will be vital to the community.

Role of School Nurses in Recovering from a Disaster

- Provide opportunities for people to come together. This will allow them to grasp the situation better.
- Provide reassurance that the crisis has passed and that students are safe.
- Openly share what information you have.
- Support parents and teachers so they can support students as they recover from the trauma.

FAST FACTS in a NUTSHELL

Disasters do happen. When or if a disaster occurs in your school, you will be a key player. Make sure you prepare in every possible way.

Clinical Snapshot

Sharon seldom is absent. When her mom became ill she needed to take several days off to care for her. Fortunately, she had oriented her substitute nurse, office secretary, and building principal well concerning her crisis plans. She was able to take off to handle her personal crisis knowing that a plan was in place in the event of a schoolwide emergency.

19

Environmental Issues

Every parent, teacher, and administrator should agree that nothing is more important than our children's health and safety, and that all children have the right to attend a school that is environmentally healthy and safe. Health and safety are intertwined; one cannot exist without the other. Learning cannot take place unless these basic needs are met.

Increasingly educators are focusing on the impact of the environment on students' health and their ability to learn. Water quality, air quality, and environmental hazards affect everyone, including a school's many occupants. The knowledge base about environmental issues continues to grow and become ever more complex.

In this chapter, you will learn:

1. Concerns about toxins and the state of school buildings today
2. The four areas of concern in the school environment, and specific toxins that may pose threats to the school environment
3. The reasons why children are more susceptible than adults to environmental toxins
4. Preventive strategies to deal with environmental toxins

ENVIRONMENTAL TOXINS

Environmental toxins have been blamed for triggering the onset of acute and chronic illnesses. Children and teachers who are ill are frequently absent, and when they are in school, they are not able to work at their full potential—learning is compromised and delayed.

The environment continues to evolve, and as we all adapt to changing circumstances, it is the job of school personnel to educate children despite any obstacles. As discussed in Chapter 1, a healthful school environment is one of the eight components of a coordinated school health program. In this area, as in many others, school nurses can play a significant role in the prevention, detection, and early correction of environmental health issues.

Healthy People 2020 Objectives

Environmental Health, 16.1

Increase the proportion of the nation's elementary, middle, and high schools that have an indoor air quality management program to promote a healthy and safe physical school environment from 51.4% in 2006 to 56.5%.

TODAY'S SCHOOL BUILDINGS

In recent years, there has been increasing concern about the conditions of school buildings. Most of these structures were built in the early 1900s with an anticipated lifespan of 50 to 100 years. These buildings have withstood decades of abuse, neglect, and conditions of terrible overcrowding. They have served generations of children well, but today many are in need of repair or replacement.

The majority of other school facilities were built in the 1960s or 1970s and had an anticipated lifespan of only about 30 years. They have also served students well but need to be repaired or to be razed and rebuilt.

Many of both types of buildings are nearing their maximum life expectancy simultaneously at a time when the nation's economy is struggling. Funding is scarce or nonexistent. The cost of building new facilities, especially with all of the new federal and state requirements, is astronomical, and repairing these outdated facilities is simply not feasible.

Unfortunately, in many cases, school buildings have not been well maintained. Tax money designated for school expenses has often gone to rising fuel and electricity costs, contracted teachers' salaries, escalating insurance costs, or newly mandated programs. School building maintenance has simply not been a priority.

When absolutely necessary, new school facilities are constructed. However, these present their own issues. The soil must be free of contaminants, the location must be away from noise, and numerous building codes must be carefully adhered to.

Consequently, school systems today are dealing with deteriorating buildings that present challenges for all kinds of health issues. As these issues are resolved, new ones continue to surface.

FAST FACTS in a NUTSHELL

Outside of home, children spend more time in school than in any other place. Many children today are enrolled in before-school care programs and often stay well beyond the regular school day for after-school care, sports, or social events. The average student spends over 14,000 total hours in school from kindergarten through grade 12.

Clinical Snapshot

Mrs. L. is concerned about her 6-year-old daughter, Lisa. Because of both parents' work schedules, Lisa participates in the before- and after-school programs, spending almost 12 hours every day in the school building. Lisa has numerous allergies to airborne toxins and various foods. Mother would like assurance from you that the prolonged school presence will not harm her child and that medical attention will be available if necessary. School nurse Ellen informs Mrs. L. that in your school, the before- and after-care program is run independently and that you are not in the building the entire time. When present, you will do all you can to protect Lisa, as you do the other children. Ellen suggests that Mrs. L speak to the before- and after-school providers and, if she is not comfortable, that she consider other child care options.

THE SCHOOL ENVIRONMENT

At a minimum, schools should be expected to have the following:

- Clean air, free from dust and mold
- Adequate climate control and ventilation
- Good air quality
- Freedom from violence
- Healthful food and clean drinking water
- No harmful bacteria or chemical dust
- Intact roofs and ceilings
- Safe stairwells and, if present, working elevators
- Well-maintained playground equipment on nontoxic soil
- Intact sidewalks, walls, and foundations
- Private, clean, working sinks; soap; and toilets

The National Association of School Nurses views the school environment as having complex interactions in four areas:

1. *Physical plant: The entire building and grounds*

Classrooms	Cafeteria
Music room	Art room
Heating system	Cooling system
Ventilation areas	Science labs
Swimming pool	Shops
Playground	Storage areas
Fields	Parking lot
Custodial areas	Hallways

2. *Occupants: Any person who enters the building or school grounds*

Staff	Parents
Students	Visitors

3. *Furnishings: All furniture, equipment, and materials in the building or on the school grounds*

Room dividers	Tables
Desks	Moving carts
Audiovisual equipment	Cleaning supplies
Chalk	Markers

| Playground equipment | Gym equipment |
| Bleachers | Sidewalks around building |

4. Activities: All activities involving personnel in the building or on the school grounds

Eating	Gym activities
Cooking	Shop work
Science lab work	Cleaning
Transportation	Field trips

SPECIFIC TOXINS

There are a wide variety of potentially threatening toxins in schools and on school property. Selekman (2006) identifies the following examples of the most common toxins, indicating where they are found and their possible effects on the body.

TABLE 19.1 Possible School Toxins

Toxin	Source	Possible Effect
Asbestos	Insulation, floor tiles	Cancer, mesothelioma
Bloodborne pathogens	Blood (nose, lacerations)	Hepatitis, AIDS
Cigarette smoke	Cigarettes, cigars	Cancer, respiratory distress
Radon	Soil	Cancer
Lead	Paint, dust, water	Delayed growth, decreased cognitive ability
Ultraviolet light	Outdoor sun exposure	Skin erythema, melanoma
Mercury	Water, equipment	Inhaled: respiratory symptoms
		Consumed: central nervous system symptoms
Solvents and other volatile organic compounds	Paint thinners, construction materials	Mucocutaneous irritation, respiratory distress

(continued)

TABLE 19.1 Possible School Toxins (*continued*)

Toxin	Source	Possible Effect
Latex	Gloves	Allergic reaction or anaphylaxis for those susceptible
Pesticides	Lice and bedbug treatments, flower and lawn care	Neurological impairment
Noise pollution	Traffic, construction	Noise-induced hearing loss
Mold and mildew	Pooled water, roof and ceiling leaks	Eye, nose, throat irritations
Classroom pets	Dander, fur, saliva, urine	Allergic reactions for those susceptible
Rodent or cockroach parts	Buildings, outside areas	Allergic reactions, asthma for those susceptible
Vehicle emissions	Running cars, school buses	Headaches, nausea, respiratory distress

Source: Seleckman (2006).

Environmentally Triggered Illnesses

These are illnesses that are reactions to common elements in a person's environment: food, chemicals, water, and tiny physical particles. Symptoms can involve multiple organs of the body, resulting in a poor state of health.

Sick-Building Syndrome

This term describes a situation in which a building occupant experiences acute symptoms linked to the time spent in the building, but no specific illness can be identified. Headaches and eye, ear, nose, and throat irritations are common. Poor ventilation or chemical contaminants are usually the cause. Symptoms subside once the person leaves the building.

CAUSES OF SUSCEPTIBILITY IN CHILDREN

Schools have become community centers. They house preschool and special needs programs, offer extended school days, and are used throughout the year. It is important now more than ever that their environments be healthy.

If you are suspicious that the school environment might be causing or exacerbating illness in your students and staff, begin to note the location, time, and symptoms displayed. Compare your notes for different parts of the building.

🔘 Clinical Snapshot

Carlos is a fifth-grade student known to have multiple airborne allergies. He frequently sees Ellen during the day with watery eyes and a sore throat. His mom reports that he does not have symptoms at home. Ellen has had no other complaints from students or parents.

Complaints of this nature should be reported to the administration and followed up with the local board of health.

Every growing child reacts differently when exposed to toxins, and children, in general, have a much lower tolerance than adults do. Sometimes, symptoms of illness can go undetected for years. Some reasons why children are more susceptible than adults are described in the following sections.

Medical Fragility

The health of children with special needs may be compromised by additional factors, such as medication use and immobility issues.

Body Size and Weight

Because children are smaller in height and weight than adults, toxins become more concentrated in their bodies. Since their body systems are developing, they are more susceptible to toxins, and extra care must be taken to provide a safe and protective school environment.

Metabolism

Children metabolize food and toxins quickly and their bodies respond rapidly.

Nutritional Status

Often, children do not eat properly. They may come to school without an adequate breakfast and have little energy in reserve. Swift and competent assessment of potential toxin exposure and appropriate follow-up care is imperative to protect children from avoidable adverse effects on their health.

Underdeveloped Immune System

Children's immune systems develop as the children do. Very young children have less, if any, immunity to foreign toxins.

Immature Brain and Central Nervous System

The nervous systems of children continue to develop as they age. Their brains are highly susceptible to assaults by foreign substances that enter their bodies.

PREVENTION STRATEGIES

As with every other aspect of health, prevention is the key. This is best accomplished through an organized preventive safety and health program. Such a program might include the following measures:

- Implementing a comprehensive school health education program in which preventive health measures (e.g., hand washing, control of communicable diseases) are taught in an organized sequential manner
- Offering annual staff education covering the recognition of anaphylaxis or any allergic responses, as well as information about bloodborne pathogens
- Insisting on the routine inspection of the building and playground equipment for structural safety
- Developing guidelines for appropriate handling of animals in the classroom
- Recommending that construction work, major cleaning, painting, and lawn services be done when the building is not occupied by students

- Setting up a proper reporting system for handling environmental concerns
- Checking to see that classrooms are clean, at a comfortable temperature, and are well ventilated
- Insisting on a no-smoking policy in the school and on the grounds
- Not permitting buses or cars to idle close to the school, where exhaust fumes can be inhaled
- Keeping careful documentation so that patterns of illnesses can be detected

ESTABLISHMENT OF LAWS AND AGENCIES DESIGNED TO PROTECT THE ENVIRONMENT

Concerns about a safe and healthy school environment have prompted the development of laws and agencies specifically designed to protect children (see Table 19.2).

TABLE 19.2 Timeline of Major Legislation and Agency Formation Established to Protect the Environment

1970	Environmental Protection Agency: Agency of the federal government charged with protecting the health and environment for all people.
1970	Occupational Safety and Health Act: Protects employees from a work environment containing health hazards.
1986	The Asbestos Hazard Emergency Response Act: Requires public and private schools to inspect school buildings for asbestos and to remove the asbestos appropriately.
1991	Occupational Safety and Health Act: Established rules to protect employees from potential exposure to blood and other body fluids.
1994	Pro-Children Act: Prohibits indoor smoking in places used to provide educational services to children younger than 18 years.

ROLE OF SCHOOL NURSES IN ENVIRONMENTAL ISSUES

- Be alert for groups of students exhibiting vague constitutional symptoms.
- Monitor, report, and intervene to correct any hazard.
- Develop Individualized Healthcare, Emergency Care, or 504 Plans to address each child's specific sensitivities.

- Have an exposure control plan in place.
- Be prepared to handle and triage a massive environmental crisis.
- Know the laws governing environmental issues in your state and district.
- Participate in committees to assess plans and implement environmental safety programs.
- Support legislation to improve environmental health.
- Offer in-service education to all staff.
- Communicate effectively with students, staff, and the administration regarding clusters of physical ailments.
- Keep detailed notes on all reports of environmental issues.
- Support school funding for construction and renovation projects.
- Be fully prepared to act in the event of an environmental emergency.

FAST FACTS in a NUTSHELL

Because of the close relationship with staff, students, parents, and members of the community, the school nurse can have a key role in prevention and early detection of harmful toxins in the school environment.

Clinical Snapshot

Ellen notes that four students and two teachers were recently diagnosed with pneumonia. All have their homerooms located in a separate wing of the building with its own forced-air heating system. Ellen reports the statistics to the building administrator, school physician, and local health department. Air quality testing may be in order.

20

Technology and the School Nurse

If today's school nurses were granted three wishes related to their jobs, they would probably be (1) less paperwork, (2) more time to spend with students, and (3) even less paperwork and even more time to spend with students. Thus far, the school nurse genie has not appeared for any of us, so we must work with what is actually available.

Technology can provide school nurses with assistance in streamlining health office paperwork. The catch is that the transition from paperwork to electronic documents will initially involve time and effort.

In this chapter, you will learn:

1. Rationale and basic uses for computers in the school health office
2. Advantages and disadvantages of a paperless health office
3. Technological equipment currently in use
4. Technical terminology
5. Steps for incorporating computers in the health office

RATIONALE

It might be helpful to keep in mind that school nursing is a specialty of the nursing profession. By definition, this means that, as professionals, school nurses continue to learn. If any of us were to see a child with an illness we had never heard of, without hesitation, we would gather information, assess the data, make a plan about how to help the patient, implement the plan, and periodically evaluate the patient and the plan for effectiveness. School nurses follow the nursing process to do their jobs effectively so that patients have good outcomes.

If school nurses lack knowledge about anything relevant to their professional performance, they must study and learn to be proficient. Computer skills are no different.

Some school nurses who began their careers without the use of computers might struggle and resist this new challenge. Those who were immediately comfortable with technology must contend with those who do not have the same level of expertise. If you are part of the first group, you must change. If you are part of the latter group, consider taking a leadership role to help your colleagues.

You have probably already developed a network of reliable resources to support you in your practice. You know whom to call for answers to certain questions. You have modeled your nursing and teaching style after those whom you admire and respect. Now you may need a technical coach to guide you. By embracing this new challenge, you will find freedom from many tedious tasks and the opportunity to spend more of your valuable time educating and helping students.

Healthy People 2020 Objectives

Health Communication and Health Information Technology, 6.1

Increase the proportion of persons with access to the Internet from 68.5% in 2007 to 75.4%.

USES OF COMPUTER TECHNOLOGY IN SCHOOL HEALTH OFFICES

There are three primary uses for computers in the health office:

1. Keeping logs (medication and daily)
2. Writing reports (monthly and annual)
3. Maintaining records (cumulative and immunization)

ADVANTAGES AND DISADVANTAGES OF A PAPERLESS HEALTH OFFICE

Most hospitals do some or all documentation electronically, and efficiently run businesses rely on technology to deliver comprehensive services to clients. Schools and their health offices are no different. Some of the advantages and disadvantages of a computerized and paperless health office are described in the following sections.

Advantages

- Information is stored, added, and easily retrieved as needed.
- Screening rosters can be printed and documents can be scanned.
- Access is limited, so privacy can be maintained.
- Tabulation of information for reports and referrals is easy.
- Memos and letters to parents can be personalized for distribution by the nurse.
- Transfer of information is easier.
- Research can be done via the Internet to reduce the number of costly reference books.
- School nurses can be quickly connected with other school nurses across the country and throughout the world.
- New school nurses can be oriented via specific teaching modules.
- Information can be accessed immediately, from any site at any time.

Disadvantages

- It can be difficult to find the exact software package to meet each nurse's needs.
- New, advanced computers are constantly being developed, and some cannot be updated.
- Training is needed, and help must be available to troubleshoot problems.
- Confidentiality remains a concern. School nurses and office personnel have an ethical responsibility to protect the integrity

of electronic student health records from both accidental and malicious tampering. Passwords are needed.
• All data must be backed up.

FAST FACTS in a NUTSHELL

You are already a savvy user of many technological devices. Now it is time to expand this knowledge to help you even more in the health office.

🔘 Clinical Snapshot

Virginia was a school nurse in a small district where she did not even have a computer. She now works in a large, urban district with other nurses with varying degrees of technical ability.

Use a team approach when dealing with technology issues. Seek in-service programs for all the nurses in your county or district and try to agree on the best program for all. This will provide continuity for transient students and as children move through the system.

ELECTRONIC EQUIPMENT CURRENTLY IN USE

Most school nurses are already technically adept to some degree. Many use the equipment described in the following sections to receive and transmit student health information.

Cell Phones and Cordless Phones

It is hard to imagine life before cell phones and cordless phones. Many school districts provide nurses with cell phones to carry with them so that they are accessible throughout the day.

Personal Digital Assistant

This is a small, battery-powered computer. Used with a stylus, similar to a small pencil, it can exchange data with another computer. Nurses like personal digital assistants because they can easily be carried in their pockets.

Voicemail

Voicemail allows people to leave messages for school nurses regarding student absences, illnesses, parental conferences, and so on. Nurses also leave voicemail messages alerting parents to concerns about their children during the school day.

Fax Machines

Fax machines and scanners are now used to transmit health information. They are most helpful in obtaining doctors' orders, parental consents, immunization dates, health records, and medication data. A health-related fax must include a cover page stating that the information being transmitted is confidential and has limited use by authorized personnel. The fax machine should be in a secure area accessible only to the school nurse and authorized staff. The nurse must be aware of any state or district policy that requires original, signed documents for doctors' orders.

FAST FACTS in a NUTSHELL

Some guidelines to keep in mind for the use of fax machines include the following:

- Fax only when time demands it.
- Send and receive only information that is necessary.
- Keep communications short.
- Remember to obtain authorization.

Clinical Snapshot

There is only one fax machine in the school building's main office. All have access to it. When sending or receiving confidential, medical information, Virginia makes sure it is marked as such and insists that no one sort these incoming faxes.

If possible, a separate fax should be provided for your exclusive use.

Answering Machines

An answering machine delivers a prerecorded message to callers and saves their messages until the school nurse listens to and deletes them. This allows the nurse to take calls when there are no other priorities.

E-Mail

It is important to have parental permission before using e-mail regarding any student. Parents must be informed that this information may be added to their child's permanent health record. There should be a confidentiality statement on all messages regarding students. For all other internal school communication, e-mail is an efficient, time-saving method of communication.

COMPUTER COMPONENTS

Computers are composed of external and internal parts. These include:

- Screen or monitor to visualize the information
- Tower containing the "brains" of the computer
- Keyboard
- Mouse—the physical object that moves and controls a pointer or display on the screen
- *Optional components:*
- Printer to transfer screen information onto paper or hardcopy
  - Removable media devices to store information
  - Compact disc
  - Flash drive

TECHNICAL TERMINOLOGY

The following information was adapted from Saugus (2009) and defines some technological terms that are commonly used.

- Boot-up—to start the computer
- Crash—unintentional shutting down of the computer

- Bug—a mistake in design of software
- Software—data or program
- Virus—a program that can harm the computer (pp. 1–8)

THE INTERNET

The Internet is the worldwide network of linked computers that provides users with access to information on the World Wide Web, as well as e-mail and file transfer services. Today's school nurse can send information and messages electronically to a parent a few blocks away sitting at his or her desk or across the world into cyberspace, the theoretical boundary of the Internet.

TELEHEALTH

Telehealth assists the school nurse in two ways. It permits the school nurse to communicate with a health care provider to discus a child's needs and attend lectures or educational programs offered where she cannot physically be present. It is especially useful in rural areas and is popular as a long-distance teaching tool.

STEPS TO CONVERT TO A COMPUTERIZED HEALTH OFFICE

The easiest, most effective method of transitioning to a computerized, paperless health office is to apply the five steps of the nursing process: data collection, assessment, planning and goal setting, implementation, and evaluation.

Data Collection

As a school nurse, one of your goals is to gain insight into your strengths and the needs of your colleagues. Start by organizing a meeting in which you all brainstorm your concerns about paperwork. Get a sense of other nurses' attitudes and abilities related to computer use.

Assessment

Review and analyze the data you have collected. Consider finances and resources that will be available to you. Discuss your concerns with any available experts: staff members of technology departments in your school district, administrators, and nurses in other districts who have already initiated programs.

Planning and Goal Setting

Set reasonable goals. Perhaps you plan to initiate a computerized program in just one school in the district. You may need to visit another health office to see how the system works. Computer and software companies sometimes send representatives to lead inservice educational programs. Check to see if you are eligible for such a program. Formulate short- and long-term plans of action.

Implementation

Carry out the initial short-term plan of action under whatever terms you have agreed upon. Try one new task at a time and do not be afraid to make a mistake. You might begin by simply printing class rosters for screening purposes or generating memos.

Evaluation

Revisit your goals to see if the actual outcome matches the intended one. If your goal was to obtain a computer for every health office and only half the offices have them, find out why. Can the situation be remedied? Perhaps the goal was to have all nurses attend a training workshop but some were not able to. Explore options for training those nurses. Reconsider the goals you made and formulate new ones to move forward.

- Accept the new challenges of technology.
- Be willing to attend workshops or take courses to learn how to use equipment.
- Seek and accept technology assistance whenever possible.
- Protect the privacy of computerized health information as you would any medical documents.

FAST FACTS in a NUTSHELL

Technology is new, different, and difficult for those who were not raised in the computer generation. It is *not* impossible to learn. Be patient with yourself. You have done harder things.

Clinical Snapshot

Virginia is a warm, caring, highly competent school nurse. She struggles with use of the computer in the health office and, intending to retire in a few years, is reluctant to learn. As a professional person who is relied upon to perform at a certain level, she must make every effort to reach out for technical knowledge and support so she can fulfill her professional obligations.

21

Top 10 Timely Troublesome Topics for the School Nurse

The greatest challenge school nurses face today may lie not with the ever-changing knowledge base or how we deliver health care but with the day-to-day situations unique to our profession. Some issues hang over school nurses, draining and depleting us of needed energy for the more important tasks involved in direct student care.

In this chapter, 10 of these frustrating issues are addressed. Certainly, there are no simple solutions for all of these problems. However, it is appropriate to share some suggestions in hopes that they will prove useful and support school nurses in recognizing that they are not alone.

TOPIC 1: LACK OF SCHOOL NURSE SUBSTITUTES

FAST FACTS in a NUTSHELL

If there is one common complaint all school nurses share, it is the lack of competent substitutes to care for students in our absence. We can assume that coverage has always been a concern, but since the passage of legislation requiring students with special needs to be placed in *the least restrictive environment*, many good, caring nurses, recognizing that greater skills would be required in the school setting, have become fearful of working independently in a school. This situation has become a crisis for many nurses and school districts.

Clinical Snapshot

School nurses shared the following experiences, describing situations in which they could not arrange for coverage:

- *Hannah came to work with a temperature of 102°F to check on a child with diabetes and give out medications.*
- *Stephanie had to miss her son's graduation.*
- *Jenna spent 15 minutes on the phone in the ER trying to find a sub while her father was experiencing chest pain.*
- *A student in Kim's school had a seizure while she was working at another school she had been sent to cover.*
- *Camila waited months for approval to attend a workshop, paid for it herself, and arranged for a sub. While standing on line at the conference registration desk, she received a call from my principal directing her to return to school immediately. The sub had cancelled.*

Suggested School Nurse Actions

A. Lobby to raise the pay for school nurse substitutes:
   - Coordinate with other districts to ensure that all substitute nurses receive pay equivalent to a per diem rate from a local agency.
   - Insist on a paid orientation for all new school nurse substitutes.
B. Recruit:
   - If some of the mothers of children in your school are registered professional nurses, and you know and trust them, ask them to consider substituting for you.
   - Call the director of nursing programs at your local university or college with bachelor's and master's programs for registered nurses and ask if any students might be interested in working as substitutes.

- Borrow a substitute from another district. If the substitute has been approved by another local board and comes with good recommendations, ask whether your board will extend the courtesy of accepting the prior board's approval so the substitute does not have to pay for another criminal background check.
- Ask the administration to add a listing seeking school nurse substitutes to any classified ad relating to employment in the district that runs in a newspaper or is posted on the district website.

C. Compromise:

- If substitute nurses cannot work the full day, have them work half days (and ask that pay be provided for the full day). Coordinate to have one work the morning and be relieved by another after lunch.

D. Make the substitute nurses' day as easy as possible:

- Do *not* leave extra work for them. Ask that they focus only on first aid.
- If health classes are scheduled, try to relieve them of this task, as well as any non-nursing tasks such as attendance or hall duty.

E. Discourage your administration from calling a nursing agency to arrange for coverage:

- Nurses provided by an agency will probably not have formal school nurse training. There will be no means to evaluate performance, and student care can be compromised.
- The district might choose to hire an emergency nurse on a full-time basis to save the cost of benefits, leaving you out of a job.

F. Remember . . .

- Your contract is with the district, *not* with a particular school. It is within the rights of the employer to send you wherever they wish. This could include covering more than one school.
- If you must travel for an emergency or more frequently, do so without complaining. Put your concerns for student safety during your absence in writing, stressing the need for your presence in one location, *not* your inconvenience.
- Do not give up trying to recruit. If one suggestion does not work, try another.

TOPIC 2: NO LUNCH, NO PREP, NO PRIVACY, AND NO ONE CARES!

FAST FACTS in a NUTSHELL

School nurses, especially if they are new and not yet certified, frequently work through the day without stopping for breaks—lunch, coffee, bathroom, or preparation times.

Clinical Snapshot

Marilyn gratefully accepted a position in a local, urban middle school with an enrollment of just over 800 students. As there were no other applicants and her two predecessors left midyear, Marilyn was given emergency certification and began immediately. Marilyn's school has five children with diabetes, 12 with anaphylaxis, two with seizure disorders, and numerous asthmatic students, as well as others with chronic diseases. Preparation time is inconceivable, nor does she *ever* have a duty-free lunch.

Frustrated one day when she is unable to make a 10-minute private call to check on her ill son, Marilyn overcomes the fear of losing her job and informs the principal that she needs uninterrupted time during the day. His response is, *I never get lunch either.*

Suggested School Nurse Actions

A. Investigate the terms of your contract. Unless the school nurse's position is addressed separately, you have the same benefits as your teacher colleagues. This includes lunch and preparation periods.

B. Attempt to work with your principal and colleagues to develop a health office schedule. Perhaps the first hours of the morning and afternoon sessions could be designated as clinic times during which nonurgent care is rendered and you see any student sent to you. The remainder of the day would be for screenings, writing, and addressing immediate needs. The quietest time of the day, usually midmorning or late afternoon, could be lunch or prep time for you.

C. Speak, in confidence, with your union representative to alert him or her of the situation. This may raise broader concerns since the teachers bargained for these rights. If they are denied you, the administration may expect others to do likewise.

D. Request additional help. Suggest the district hire a registered professional nurse to work on an hourly basis for even 1 or 2 hours a day. Emphasize that this nurse would also be someone comfortable covering in your absence and the cost would be minimal. Stress the safety factor in having adequate coverage for the school's medically fragile students. If this nurse is competent, encourage her or him to consider pursuing additional preparation to become a school nurse. Offer to help the nurse reach this goal.

TOPIC 3: HEALTH CARE REFORM

FAST FACTS in a NUTSHELL

The Centers for Disease Control and Prevention (CDC) reported that the percentage of children without health insurance was 8.9% in 2008 (CDC, 2009). This equated to approximately 1 child out of every 11 who did not have medical benefits.

Clinical Snapshot
School nurse Debbie is competent and caring but was unaware that one student's dad had lost his job, leaving the family without health benefits. The student has a chronic disease that requires medical management and long-term drug therapy. Debbie should be aware of this family's temporary needs and refer them to agencies for help in finding appropriate medical care.

The Affordable Care Act passed in March 2010 and implemented in January 2014 was designed to allow consumers greater control of their health care. It includes the Patient Bill of Rights, which now gives the American people the stability and flexibility they need to make informed choices about their health.

One aspect of this Act is that health plans can no longer limit or deny benefits to children under 19 years of age because of preexisting conditions (U.S. Department of Health and Human Services, n.d.).

Suggested School Nurse Actions

A. Familiarize yourself with the families of your students, especially those with extensive medical needs, unemployment issues, or a transient lifestyle.

B. Question parents about health care coverage.

C. Help link parents with services and rights to which they are entitled under the law.

D. Seek to make available donations of cash or food gift cards for families in need, no questions asked.

E. Consider participating in community projects to help stock local food pantries.

TOPIC 4: SCHOOL-SPONSORED BEFORE- AND AFTER-CARE PROGRAMS, ACTIVITIES, AND CLASS TRIPS

FAST FACTS in a NUTSHELL

Today's school day is quite different than that of the past. With so many working and single-parent homes, a significant number of children begin their day hours before the first class and stay in the building well into the evening. Class field trips are commonly scheduled every year and all students participate. Those with special needs must be cared for by a registered professional nurse before and after school, and while attending class trips.

Clinical Snapshot

Theresa had planned to stay late to finish up some paperwork. For 2 hours as she tries to complete this work, she is repeatedly interrupted by students who are involved in after-school sports, others who are in the after-school program, and parents who want to visit when they come to pick up their child. Theresa is tempted to take some of the charts home to work on but resists the impulse, knowing that student health records are legal documents that should not leave the school.

Most districts have some plan to meet the needs of single parents and those whose workday extends beyond the normal school hours. Programs are offered that enable students to begin their day before the first class and extend into the early evening. Know the particulars of those that are independently run and those that are sponsored by the school.

Many schools also offer sports or extracurricular activities outside of the school day. For the school nurse, this means that she or he is virtually never in the building without children or staff present. If no substitute nurse is available to go on a field trip to administer medication, then the school nurse must go. This means the rest of the school is left with no coverage.

Suggested School Nurse Actions

A. Review the protocol of providers who coordinate before- or after-care programs or other school events. If the program is not school sponsored and the care provider does not offer nursing coverage, make sure parents are aware of this.
B. Speak with your principal and have him or her stress to staff that you should not be depended on for care outside of school hours.
C. Check with your union leaders to clarify your responsibilities if you are in the building off hours.
D. Try not to get caught while you are sitting or standing behind your desk. When a parent or staff member approaches and you do not have time to speak, greet them at your door or in the hallway. You can then excuse yourself and walk away without appearing rude.
E. If students with medical needs are participating in after-school sports, try to have a coach trained as a delegate for epinephrine or glucagon use.
F. If you are working before or after school hours, close your door and hide! Let no one know you are working. If there is a *true* emergency, they will find you, and for this occasional instance, you will certainly not mind being interrupted.

School-Sponsored Trips

In most schools, children go on a yearly class trip. It would be hurtful and possibly illegal to exclude a student from these activities because of a special need or lack of money. If a child in that class needs medication or a specific treatment, a nurse must accompany the class wherever they go. This presents a problem as a substitute nurse must be provided, either to go on the trip or to cover the school so you can go.

Suggested School Nurse Actions

A. In planning class trips, check to see whether a parent of the child with medical needs can attend. Have the teacher plan well in advance so parents have ample time to arrange their schedules.
B. See Topic 1, earlier, regarding suggestions for obtaining substitute nurses.
C. Investigate the possibility of keeping a small amount of money available to cover the costs for students who cannot afford to go on trips (or any other pressing need you are aware of). The names of those who access this money must be kept in confidence. Seek funding from the parent–teacher association or any group willing to trust your judgment.
D. If a child requires the use of epinephrine due to food allergies, check to see if a trained delegate may be permitted to go on the field trip in lieu of a substitute registered nurse.

TOPIC 5: MEDICALLY FRAGILE STUDENTS NEEDING ONE-ON-ONE CARE

Suggested School Nurse Actions

A. Participate in making the assessment of needs and recommending the level of care that the student with medical needs receives—health aide, licensed practical nurse, or registered nurse.
B. Meet with the child, parents, and other Child Study Team members to perform the evaluation properly before the child is placed in class. You do *not* need to be part of the discussion of who pays for this service.
C. At the first meeting raise the question of who carries full responsibility for the child's care. If the caregiver is an aide or a licensed practical nurse, you, as the certified school nurse, may

Today we recognize that children with chronic diseases or conditions are part of the mainstream. Bear in mind that the Individuals with Disabilities Education Act (IDEA, 1990) states that all children are entitled to *a free and public education in the least restrictive environment.* Some of these children are considered *nursing dependent* or *medically fragile* and may be *technology dependent* as well (Washington State model).

Clinical Snapshop

Mary is fortunate that there is a competent nurse assigned to her nursing-dependent student. However, when the nurse is absent or problems arise, Mary must be prepared to intervene. The overwhelming accommodations needed for these special children can compromise Mary's available time for the remaining students.

be in charge. Put your questions and responses in writing or make sure the discussion is part of the minutes for the meeting.

D. Clarify who is to care for the child if the designated individual is absent. If you are expected to step in, request that your office be covered by a substitute nurse.

E. Get to know the child and his or her needs. Even if one-on-one care is provided, the child is still your student.

F. Get to know the one-on-one provider. Check to be sure someone is evaluating him or her.

TOPIC 6: PROFESSIONAL RESPONSIBILITIES

Suggested School Nurse Actions

A. *Before* any meeting you plan to attend, clarify who is to determine if you should be interrupted. A busy secretary might not want her work interrupted or may feel it is not her job to care for sick children.

B. Come to a mutual agreement with the administrator and secretary about what is expected in your absence and what constitutes an emergency.

Administrators are sometimes reluctant to include you in meetings that require you to be out of your office as it means someone must cover your calls and office visits and, realistically, no one wants to do this.

Clinical Snapshot

The director of special services has requested Tanya's presence at a Child Study Team meeting to assess the level of care necessary for a medically fragile child who will be attending her school. As the school nurse, Tanya researches the child's condition, reads the medical records, visits the child at home, sees the student in the current school placement, and speaks with the parents in preparation for the meeting.

Tanya informs the principal that she will be out of her office for the designated meeting time, yet she is called by the secretary to return to your office twice—first for a child who wet his pants and next for a child who was tired.

C. Clarify who is in charge. If the director of special services or any administrator requires your participation in a meeting, the secretary should not be overriding the director's decision by summoning you out of the meeting for a nonemergency.

D. When discussing your professional performance with the administration, stress that the priorities of your tasks should be to *do what no other staff member can do*, not what the other staff member *chooses not to do*.

E. Do not accept the rationale that there is no one else who is available to help. In many cases, insisting on having a nurse to handle a situation is the path of least resistance. Rather than confronting the other staff member, administrators may continue to let non-nursing tasks fall on you because you will get the job done. However, you cannot be in two places at the same time, have numerous bosses, or remain excluded from participating in educational or medical planning that requires your input or for which only you are qualified.

F. Review your contract to see what rights the other teachers and staff members are given. If they are entitled to duty-free lunch and prep periods, you should be, too.

G. Accept that there may be times when your constant presence in the building will be necessary for the well-being of certain students. This is the nature of the beast. Investigate additional compensation, other local nurses who could cover, or a rotating nurse to cover all nurse lunches in the district.

TOPIC 7: UNLICENSED OR NONCERTIFIED PERSONNEL IN THE HEALTH OFFICE

=========== *FAST FACTS in a NUTSHELL*

Ideally, every school should have *at least* one nurse who is certified in the specialty of school nursing.

Clinical Snapshot

Today's school health office is a busy place. When the enrollment is large or student needs are complex, health aides or health assistants, may be necessary. These registered nurses provide needed help to the school nurse and are most welcome.

The problem arises when a district, often in an attempt to save money, permits a nurse who has had no preparation or experience as a school nurse to work independently. Frequently, the certified school nurse must serve as the supervisor for a noncertified nurse working in another building. The certified nurse may be legally responsible for the noncertified nurse's job performance.

Suggested School Nurse Actions

A. As positions arise within your district, encourage your administration to hire only properly credentialed nurses. When it comes to the health and safety of children, money should not be an issue.
B. All personnel must have a clearly written job description that does *not* conflict with the role of the certified school nurse. Check with your administration and union officials to make sure there is no confusion before a conflict arises.

C. If the district is unionized, the school nurse should be included in the contract. That means he or she pays dues as do the teachers and is entitled to be placed on salary guide and receive the same rights and benefits.

D. Secretaries or administrative assistants are a valuable help to the school nurse. They can handle phone calls, order supplies, and perform clerical tasks while working within their job description. They should *not* be involved in assessing students, conferencing with staff or parents, attending meetings on behalf of the school nurse, charting, or giving medications.

TOPIC 8: SCHOOL NURSE SUPERVISION AND EVALUATION; STUDENT GROWTH OBJECTIVES

FAST FACTS in a NUTSHELL

All schools have some type of evaluation process for professional staff. Unfortunately, school nurses are seldom evaluated by an administrator who truly understands what we do. Some districts are now using nationally recognized programs that provide a generic outline of items to be considered in evaluation.

Clinical Snapshot

Isabella has been a school nurse for more than 20 years. She has had nothing but glowing evaluations from every administrator. However, no one has ever offered her constructive suggestions to better her practice.

Student growth objectives (SGOs) are the latest initiative introduced in some states to assess and improve student instruction. As a school nurse, you are considered a support specialist and may be obligated to partake in the requirements.

Suggested School Nurse Actions

A. Investigate the evaluation tool your district is using. If this tool is comprehensive, valid, and reflects what you do, accept it.

B. If you have questions on the effectiveness of the evaluation tool, raise your concerns *before* you are evaluated. Once the evaluation is completed, you will have little chance to have it altered.

C. Consider obtaining administrative or supervisory certification yourself so that you can evaluate other school nurses. It would be more beneficial if our evaluations contained constructive suggestions for improvement from a knowledgeable source.

D. If you have been told you must write SGOs, the objectives you have previously identified for your own practice might serve as a guide. You might wish to spend less time on non-nursing tasks or have all your Individualized Healthcare Plans (IHPs) completed by a certain date. You can also work with colleagues to formulate district-wide objectives.

E. Find your own school nurse role model to guide you to a better nursing practice. We all can improve in some way.

TOPIC 9: PEDICULOSIS

===*FAST FACTS in a NUTSHELL*

The American Association of Pediatrics and the National Association of School Nurses (NASN) agree that no-nit policies in schools should be discontinued (NASN, 2011a).

Clinical Snapshot

School nurse Anna spends the entire month of September looking through children's heads for lice. The nurse who preceded her told her this was expected.

Head lice are probably responsible for more wasted school nurse hours than any other issue. Teachers panic, administrators do not know what to do, and parents will drive you insane when a child is identified with pediculosis. School nurses know that lice cause no threat to health, are nothing more than a nuisance, and, in terms of protecting students from illness, our time would be better spent doing a daily temperature check on every student.

Children found to have head lice should remain in class but be discouraged from close direct head contact with others. The educational process should not be disrupted (NASN, 2011a).

Suggested School Nurse Actions

A. Research your school policy. If you have a no-nit policy, seek to change it *before* there are reported cases to deal with. Education is the key here and it cannot be provided effectively in the middle of an outbreak. Educate before the problem manifests, when parents, staff, and administration are more receptive.

B. If a case is reported, check that student and his or her siblings. If several cases are seen in the same class, check the entire class. Mass schoolwide screenings are *not* necessary. Check students at the end of the school day. This way if a case is detected, the child will be going home shortly and it will not be necessary to embarrass him or her by summoning a parent from work for an early dismissal. Notify the parent by phone. Check the student the following day to be sure he or she has been treated, and allow the child to return. Refer parents to a physician for information about the best treatment product, as you would with any other disease.

C. Send a notice home in September regarding all communicable diseases (streptococcal infections, viruses, impetigo, coxsackie, conjunctivitis, lice, etc.). List the symptoms to watch for and explain that these diseases are commonly seen in school-aged children. For the parents who *insist* that a notice about communicable diseases be sent home, *you have already done it!* This notice early in the school year is also a good time to remind parents to keep the ill children at home and send a note upon return, and to clarify when a physician's clearance is required for return to school.

D. With administrative approval, consider sending a separate notice home only if you have numerous cases of lice or any other disease.

E. Refuse to disclose the names of infected children. Suggest that parents notify the playmates of affected children.

TOPIC 10: PRIORITIZING TASKS

Suggested School Nurse Actions

A. **Contact Information**
   • Make sure every adult and child in the building has a current emergency card that is completed, signed, and available in your office.

Always put the needs of the students first. Reports, charting, administrative demands, meetings, phone calls, and so on, can all wait.

Clinical Snapshot

Olivia has finished her required school nurse course work and has landed her long-anticipated job. Now she is overwhelmed by the numerous tasks before her. She takes a deep breath, relaxes, and starts to prioritize what must be done immediately and what can be put temporarily on the back burner.

Students
- Do not discard the previous year's cards; you may need to refer to them for additional phone contacts. Include a section that parents can use for updating any recent health concerns involving their child.

Faculty and Staff
- Include a few blank lines that the teacher can initial for the next year if there are no changes or use for updating any new issues.

B. Children with Special Needs

Identify
- Review health data for each child: physical exams, former school records, medications, restrictions, treatments, and so on.
- Place the information in individual folders
- Ask the previous school nurse, secretary, and teachers to share any health information with you.
- Contact each parent or guardian to request updated information.
- Obtain written permission to share information with those who have a need to know.

Develop List
- Write a confidential list, for your use only, of all children with special needs.
- Meet with every child's teacher and share what and with whom you have been given permission to share.
- Do not distribute copies of the list.

Recordkeeping
- Write IHPs and Emergency Care Plans (ECPs) for those in need.
- Use reference books or software programs to develop a standard format for these plans.
- Check to see if your colleagues have IHPs they would be willing to share, and adapt them for your students. If there are no changes from the previous year, you and the child's parents can just sign off on the prior year's plan for the upcoming year.

C. Medications
Identify
- Check to be sure you have medications for all children who *need* to be dosed during the school day. You will want to have the medication, along with the permission slips from the parent and physician, on hand before the child starts school. Check expiration dates, physician's orders, and parental consents.

Develop List
- Write down the names of those children needing daily medications and those with "prn" orders.
- Create a binder or computer-generated portfolio with separate charting sheets for each child.

Recordkeeping
- Chart immediately after each dose is given.

Tips
- Give medication only to the child whose name is indicated on the container—no sharing.
- Count controlled medications with the adult who brings them in.
- Insist that all medications be provided in their original containers.
- Keep all medications locked, except those needed for emergency administration.
- Have a stock nebulizer, tubing, and epinephrine available.
- Place epinephrine and glucagon in a safe, secure, unlocked location.
- Check delegates training form indicating specific child.
- Attach each child's ECP and contact information with his or medication.

D. Immunizations
Identify
- Make an outline of all the state-required immunizations and post it on your desk for immediate reference.

- Get an updated list of the entire school population according to class or grade.
- Have a health folder for every student, including those placed out of district.
- Review all immunization dates, comparing the time sequence with the birth date.

Develop List

- Prepare a form that you can use as a checklist to ensure that all required health documents and immunizations have been received. Include the student's name, birth date, date of last physical exam, and so on.
- Send the form out to parents of children whose records are incomplete, indicating what is needed, and give a deadline for submission.
- Keep a list of those students who are deficient in immunizations.
- If the response from parents is not timely, send second notice, and copy your administrator.
- If the parents still do not respond, ask your administrator to intervene and threaten exclusion.

Recordkeeping

- For those whose records appear complete, place information in the child's folder to be filled in at a later date.

E. Standing Orders

Identify

- Identify the procedures you and the school physician feel are appropriate for delivering health care to students. If you do not have standing orders, ask colleagues in neighboring districts if they will share theirs and adapt them for your district.

Develop List

- Review the standing orders carefully and make changes as needed. You may only order supplies included in your standing orders.

Recordkeeping

- Review and have the orders signed annually by the school physician. This is best done in June in preparation for the following school year.

Appendix C contains a month-by-month suggested outline of tasks, which will give you further insight into what must be done immediately.

Healthy People 2020 Topics

A

Access to Health Services
Adolescent Health (*New*)
Arthritis, Osteoporosis, and
    Chronic Back Conditions

B

Blood Disorders and Blood
    Safety (*New*)

C

Cancer
Chronic Kidney Disease

D

Dementias, Including Alzheim-
    er's Disease (*New*)
Diabetes
Disability and Health

E

Early and Middle Childhood
    (*New*)
Educational and Community-
    Based Programs
Environmental Health

F

Family Planning
Food Safety

G

Genomics (*New*)
Global Health (*New*)

H

Health Communication
    and Health Information
    Technology

Healthcare-Associated Infections (*New*)

Health-Related Quality of Life and Well-Being (*New*)

Hearing and Other Sensory or Communication Disorders

Heart Disease and Stroke

HIV

I

Immunization and Infectious Diseases

Injury and Violence Prevention

L

Lesbian, Gay, Bisexual, and Transgender Health (*New*)

M

Maternal, Infant, and Child Health

Medical Product Safety

Mental Health and Mental Disorders

N

Nutrition and Weight Status

O

Occupational Safety and Health

Older Adults (*New*)

Oral Health

P

Physical Activity

Preparedness (*New*)

Public Health Infrastructure

R

Respiratory Diseases

S

Sexually Transmitted Diseases

Sleep Health (*New*)

Social Determinants of Health (*New*)

Substance Abuse

T

Tobacco Use

V

Vision

Adapted from Healthy People 2020. (n.d.). Topics and Objectives—Objectives A–Z. U.S. Department of Health and Human Services. Retrieved August 10, 2014 from www.healthypeople.gov/2020/topicsobjectives2020/

B

Health Office Set-Up

FIRST-AID SUPPLIES

- Bandages
- Ice packs
- Arm and leg splints
- Soap and other antiseptics
- Paper towels

EQUIPMENT

- Privacy screen
- File cabinet
- Desk
- Swivel chair
- Cot with paper roll
- Double-lock medicine cabinet
- Dedicated phone line
- Refrigerator large enough for medications and ice packs
- Several chairs
- Air conditioner
- Computer

ASSESSMENT TOOLS

- Several types of thermometers
- Blood pressure machine with adult and pediatric cuffs
- Stethoscope

- Audiometer
- Vision testing equipment
- Scoliometer
- Height, growth, and basal metabolic index (BMI) charts
- Scale

BATHROOM

- Window or exhaust system
- Doorway wide enough to permit wheelchair access
- Sink with eyewash station

Month-by-Month Calendar of Tasks

*AUGUST

1. Unpack supplies. Clean and prepare the office for the first day of school.
2. Review information on incoming students. Set up charts.
3. Send written notices or make phone calls if deficiencies are found in examination or immunization records.
4. Note students with specific medical needs.
5. Formulate a student-alert list for your own reference. Do not disseminate it to staff.
6. Check standing orders. Update as needed.
7. Review individualized health care plans and emergency health plans from the previous year. Write plans for new students.
8. Check students who receive medication in school; review physician orders, parental consents, asthma action plans, and so on.
9. Contact parents who have children with severe allergies, asthma, or seizure disorders. Get medications and paperwork *before* students enter school.
10. Check expiration dates on all medications.
11. Check locks on medication and supply cabinets.
12. Prepare plans for substitute nurses.
13. Formulate goals for the new school year.

*Look into getting paid for these noncontractual hours. If other members of the Child Study Team are compensated, you may be entitled also.

SEPTEMBER

1. Have students' folders arranged by class or grade level.
2. Make sure all students have had state-required immunizations. File an immunization status report if it is required by your state.
3. Meet individually with teachers to review students' health needs.
4. Introduce yourself to new students, teachers, and parents.
5. Distribute, collect, and review emergency information for students and staff.
6. Conduct a staff in-service education program covering Heimlich maneuver, automated external defibrillator (AED), glucagon, and epinephrine autoinjector. Distribute universal precaution supplies.
7. Check on staff certifications for cardiopulmonary resuscitation and automated external defibrillator use. Arrange renewals as needed.
8. Organize epinephrine autoinjector and glucagon delegates, and have consent forms signed. Do training.
9. Begin tuberculosis testing.
10. Review team assignments: Crisis, 504, Intervention and Referral, Child Study.
11. Review previous year's goals, student growth outcomes, professional improvement plans. Formulate new ones.
12. Health folder check. Review each class list making sure you have a folder for every child.

OCTOBER

1. Begin screenings: height and weight.
2. Start blood pressure screenings.

NOVEMBER

1. Review and update individual health care and emergency plans.
2. Continue screenings: vision and hearing.

DECEMBER

1. Continue screenings: vision and hearing.

JANUARY

1. Continue screenings: vision and hearing.
2. Review documentation for all students: check immunizations, referrals, deficiencies, care plans, medications, and so on.

FEBRUARY

1. Continue screenings: dental and blood pressure.
2. Check outdoor playground equipment for damage from winter months.

MARCH

1. Screenings: basal metabolic index (BMI).
2. Conduct kindergarten registration. Review incoming students' records.

APRIL

1. Screenings: scoliosis.
2. Review goals for the school year. Begin to formulate new goals for the upcoming year.

MAY

1. Begin charting screening results. Follow up on all outstanding referrals.
2. Review and update standing orders.
3. Order supplies for the new school year.
4. Make teacher recommendations for students with special needs.

JUNE

1. Prepare an annual report.
2. Close out documentation and transfer information to sending schools.
3. Notify parents to obtain medications. Send medication permission slips out for the coming school year. Return unused medications to parents.

4. Have standing orders signed by the school physician to cover the upcoming school year.
5. Dispose of medical waste (e.g., sharps) according to district policy.
6. Review records of incoming students, inform parents of deficiencies, and set up folders.
7. Transfer records and give verbal reports on outgoing students to receiving nurses.
8. Do a supply inventory. Order supplies as needed.
9. Prepare an annual report.
10. Send notices for students requiring physical examinations in September.
11. Send equipment out for calibration.

Recommended Immunizations, 2014

APPENDIX D1

2014 Recommended Immunizations for Children from Birth Through 6 Years Old

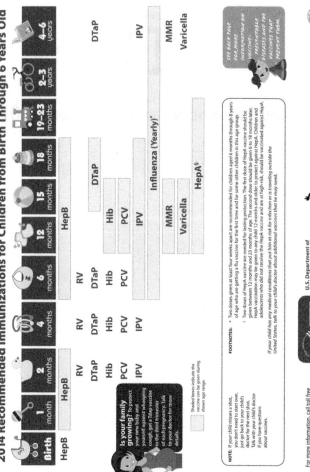

Is your family growing? To protect your new baby and yourself against whooping cough, get a Tdap vaccine in the third trimester of each pregnancy. Talk to your doctor for more details.

Shaded boxes indicate the vaccine can be given during shown age range.

NOTE: If your child misses a shot, you don't need to start over, just go back to your child's doctor for the next shot. Talk with your child's doctor if you have questions about vaccines.

FOOTNOTES:

* Two doses given at least four weeks apart are recommended for children aged 6 months through 8 years of age who are getting a flu vaccine for the first time and for some other children in this age group.

‡ Two doses of HepA vaccine are needed for lasting protection. The first dose of HepA vaccine should be given between 12 months and 23 months of age. The second dose should be given 6 to 18 months later. HepA vaccination may be given to any child 12 months and older to protect against HepA. Children and adolescents who did not receive the HepA vaccine and are at high-risk, should be vaccinated against HepA.

If your child has any medical conditions that put him at risk for infection or is traveling outside the United States, talk to your child's doctor about additional vaccines that he may need.

For more information, call toll free
1-800-CDC-INFO (1-800-232-4636)
or visit
http://www.cdc.gov/vaccines

U.S. Department of Health and Human Services
Centers for Disease Control and Prevention

AMERICAN ACADEMY OF FAMILY PHYSICIANS
STRONG MEDICINE FOR AMERICA

American Academy of Pediatrics
DEDICATED TO THE HEALTH OF ALL CHILDREN

Vaccine-Preventable Diseases and the Vaccines that Prevent Them

Disease	Vaccine	Disease spread by	Disease symptoms	Disease complications
Chickenpox	Varicella vaccine protects against chickenpox.	Air, direct contact	Rash, tiredness, headache, fever	Infected blisters, bleeding disorders, encephalitis (brain swelling), pneumonia (infection in the lungs)
Diphtheria	DTaP* vaccine protects against diphtheria.	Air, direct contact	Sore throat, mild fever, weakness, swollen glands in neck	Swelling of the heart muscle, heart failure, coma, paralysis, death
Hib	Hib vaccine protects against *Haemophilus influenzae* type b.	Air, direct contact	May be no symptoms unless bacteria enter the blood	Meningitis (infection of the covering around the brain and spinal cord), intellectual disability, epiglottitis (life-threatening infection that can block the windpipe and lead to serious breathing problems), pneumonia (infection in the lungs), death
Hepatitis A	HepA vaccine protects against hepatitis A.	Direct contact, contaminated food or water	May be no symptoms, fever, stomach pain, loss of appetite, fatigue, vomiting, jaundice (yellowing of skin and eyes), dark urine	Liver failure, arthralgia (joint pain), kidney, pancreatic, and blood disorders
Hepatitis B	HepB vaccine protects against hepatitis B.	Contact with blood or body fluids	May be no symptoms, fever, headache, weakness, vomiting, jaundice (yellowing of skin and eyes), joint pain	Chronic liver infection, liver failure, liver cancer
Flu	Flu vaccine protects against influenza.	Air, direct contact	Fever, muscle pain, sore throat, cough, extreme fatigue	Pneumonia (infection in the lungs)
Measles	MMR** vaccine protects against measles.	Air, direct contact	Rash, fever, cough, runny nose, pinkeye	Encephalitis (brain swelling), pneumonia (infection in the lungs), death
Mumps	MMR** vaccine protects against mumps.	Air, direct contact	Swollen salivary glands (under the jaw), fever, headache, tiredness, muscle pain	Meningitis (infection of the covering around the brain and spinal cord), encephalitis (brain swelling), inflammation of testicles or ovaries, deafness
Pertussis	DTaP* vaccine protects against pertussis (whooping cough).	Air, direct contact	Severe cough, runny nose, apnea (a pause in breathing in infants)	Pneumonia (infection in the lungs), death
Polio	IPV vaccine protects against polio.	Air, direct contact, through the mouth	May be no symptoms, sore throat, fever, nausea, headache	Paralysis, death
Pneumococcal	PCV vaccine protects against pneumococcus.	Air, direct contact	May be no symptoms, pneumonia (infection in the lungs)	Bacteremia (blood infection), meningitis (infection of the covering around the brain and spinal cord), death
Rotavirus	RV vaccine protects against rotavirus.	Through the mouth	Diarrhea, fever, vomiting	Severe diarrhea, dehydration
Rubella	MMR** vaccine protects against rubella.	Air, direct contact	Children infected with rubella virus sometimes have a rash, fever, swollen lymph nodes	Very serious in pregnant women—can lead to miscarriage, stillbirth, premature delivery, birth defects
Tetanus	DTaP* vaccine protects against tetanus.	Exposure through cuts in skin	Stiffness in neck and abdominal muscles, difficulty swallowing, muscle spasms, fever	Broken bones, breathing difficulty, death

* DTaP combines protection against diphtheria, tetanus, and pertussis.
** MMR combines protection against measles, mumps, and rubella.

Last updated January 2014 • CS245366-A

APPENDIX D2

2014 Recommended Immunizations for Children from 7 Through 18 Years Old

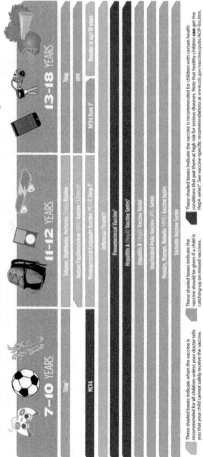

7–10 YEARS	11–12 YEARS	13–18 YEARS
Tdap[1]	Tetanus, Diphtheria, Pertussis (Tdap) Vaccine[1]	Tdap
	Human Papillomavirus (HPV) Vaccine (3 Doses)[2]	HPV
MCV4	Meningococcal Conjugate Vaccine MCV4 Dose 1[3]	MCV4 Dose 1[3] Booster at age 16 years
	Influenza (Yearly)	
	Pneumococcal Vaccine[5]	
	Hepatitis A (HepA) Vaccine Series[6]	
	Hepatitis B (HepB) Vaccine Series	
	Inactivated Polio Vaccine (IPV) Series	
	Measles, Mumps, Rubella (MMR) Vaccine Series	
	Varicella Vaccine Series	

These boxes indicate when the vaccine is recommended for all children unless your doctor tells you that your child cannot safely receive the vaccine.

These shaded boxes indicate the vaccine should be given if a child is catching-up on missed vaccines.

These shaded boxes indicate the vaccine is recommended for children with certain health conditions that put them at high risk for serious diseases. Note that healthy children can get the HepA series.* See vaccine-specific recommendations at www.cdc.gov/vaccines/pubs/ACIP-list.htm.

FOOTNOTES

[1] Tdap vaccine is combination vaccine that is recommended at age 11 or 12 to protect against tetanus, diphtheria and pertussis. If your child has not received any or all of the DTaP vaccine series, or if you don't know if your child has received these shots, your child needs a single dose of Tdap when they are 7-10 years old. Talk to your child's health care provider to find out if they need additional catch-up vaccines.

[2] All 11 or 12 year olds—both girls and boys—should receive 3 doses of HPV vaccine to protect against HPV-related disease. Either HPV vaccine (Cervarix® or Gardasil®) can be given to girls and young women; only one HPV vaccine (Gardasil®) can be given to boys and young men.

[3] Meningococcal conjugate vaccine (MCV) is recommended at age 11 or 12. A booster shot is recommended at age 16. Teens who received MCV for the first time at age 13 through 15 years will need a one-time booster dose between the ages of 16 and 18 years. If your teenager missed getting the vaccine altogether, ask their health care provider about getting it now, especially if your teenager is about to move into a college dorm or military barracks.

[4] Everyone 6 months of age and older—including preteens and teens—should get a flu vaccine every year. Children under the age of 9 years may require more than one dose. Talk to your child's health care provider to find out if they need more than one dose.

[5] Pneumococcal Conjugate Vaccine (PCV13) and Pneumococcal Polysaccharide Vaccine (PPSV23) are recommended for some children through 18 years old with certain medical conditions that place them at high risk. Talk to your healthcare provider about pneumococcal vaccines and what factors may place your child at high risk for pneumococcal disease.

[6] Hepatitis A vaccination is recommended for older children with certain medical conditions that place them at high risk. HepA vaccine is licensed, safe, and effective for all children of all ages. Even if your child is not at high risk, you may decide you want your child protected against HepA. Talk to your healthcare provider about HepA vaccine and what factors may place your child at high risk for HepA.

For more information, call toll free 1-800-CDC-INFO (1-800-232-4636) or visit http://www.cdc.gov/vaccines/teens

CDC

U.S. Department of Health and Human Services
Centers for Disease Control and Prevention

American Academy of Pediatrics
DEDICATED TO THE HEALTH OF ALL CHILDREN™

AMERICAN ACADEMY OF FAMILY PHYSICIANS
STRONG MEDICINE FOR AMERICA

Vaccine-Preventable Diseases and the Vaccines that Prevent Them

Diphtheria *(Can be prevented by Tdap vaccine)*

Diphtheria is a very contagious bacterial disease that affects the respiratory system, including the lungs. Diphtheria bacteria can be passed from person to person by direct contact with droplets from an infected person's cough or sneeze. When people are infected, the diphtheria bacteria produce a toxin (poison) in the body that can cause weakness, sore throat, low-grade fever, and swollen glands in the neck. Effects from this toxin can also lead to swelling of the heart muscle and, in some cases, heart failure. In severe cases, the illness can cause coma, paralysis, and even death.

Hepatitis A *(Can be prevented by HepA vaccine)*

Hepatitis A is an infection in the liver caused by hepatitis A virus. The virus is spread primarily person-to-person through the fecal-oral route. In other words, the virus is taken in by mouth from contact with objects, food, or drinks contaminated by the feces (stool) of an infected person. Symptoms include fever, tiredness, loss of appetite, nausea, abdominal discomfort, dark urine, and jaundice (yellowing of the skin and eyes). An infected person may have no symptoms, may have mild illness for a week or two, or may have severe illness for several months that requires hospitalization. In the U.S., about 100 people a year die from hepatitis A.

Hepatitis B *(Can be prevented by HepB vaccine)*

Hepatitis B is an infection of the liver caused by hepatitis B virus. The virus spreads through exchange of blood or other body fluids, for example, from sharing personal items, such as razors or during sex. Hepatitis B causes a flu-like illness with loss of appetite, nausea, vomiting, rashes, joint pain, and jaundice. The virus stays in the liver of some people for the rest of their lives and can result in severe liver diseases, including fatal cancer.

Human Papillomavirus *(Can be prevented by HPV vaccine)*

Human papillomavirus is a common virus. HPV is most common in people in their teens and early 20s. It is the major cause of cervical cancer in women and genital warts in women and men. The strains of HPV that cause cervical cancer and genital warts are spread during sex.

Influenza *(Can be prevented by annual flu vaccine)*

Influenza is a highly contagious viral infection of the nose, throat, and lungs. The virus spreads easily through droplets when an infected person coughs or sneezes and can cause mild to severe illness. Typical symptoms include a sudden high fever, chills, a dry cough, headache, runny nose, sore throat, and muscle and joint pain. Extreme fatigue can last from several days to weeks. Influenza may lead to hospitalization or even death, even among previously healthy children.

Measles *(Can be prevented by MMR vaccine)*

Measles is one of the most contagious viral diseases. Measles virus is spread by direct contact with the airborne respiratory droplets of an infected person. Measles is so contagious that just being in the same room after a person who has measles has already left can result in infection. Symptoms usually include a rash, fever, cough, and red, watery eyes. Fever can persist, rash can last for up to a week, and coughing can last about 10 days. Measles can also cause pneumonia, seizures, brain damage, or death.

Meningococcal Disease *(Can be prevented by MCV vaccine)*

Meningococcal disease is caused by bacteria and is a leading cause of bacterial meningitis (infection around the brain and spinal cord) in children. The bacteria are spread through the exchange of nose and throat droplets, such as when coughing, sneezing or kissing. Symptoms include nausea, vomiting, sensitivity to light, confusion and sleepiness. Meningococcal disease also causes blood infections. About one of every ten people who get the disease dies from it. Survivors of meningococcal disease may lose their arms or legs, become deaf, have problems with their nervous systems, become developmentally disabled, or suffer seizures or strokes.

Mumps *(Can be prevented by MMR vaccine)*

Mumps is an infectious disease caused by the mumps virus, which is spread in the air by a cough or sneeze from an infected person. A child can also get infected with mumps by coming in contact with a contaminated object, like a toy. The mumps virus causes fever, headaches, painful swelling of the salivary glands under the jaw, fever, muscle aches, tiredness, and loss of appetite. Severe complications for children who get mumps are uncommon, but can include meningitis (infection of the covering of the brain and spinal cord), encephalitis (inflammation of the brain), permanent hearing loss, or swelling of the testes, which rarely can lead to sterility in men.

Pertussis *(Whooping Cough) (Can be prevented by Tdap vaccine)*

Pertussis is caused by bacteria spread through direct contact with respiratory droplets when an infected person coughs or sneezes. In the beginning, symptoms of pertussis are similar to the common cold, including runny nose, sneezing, and cough. After 1-2 weeks, pertussis can cause spells of violent coughing and choking, making it hard to breathe, drink, or eat. This cough can last for weeks. Pertussis is most serious for babies, who can get pneumonia, have seizures, become brain damaged, or even die. About two-thirds of children under 1 year of age who get pertussis must be hospitalized.

Pneumococcal Disease

(Can be prevented by Pneumococcal vaccine)

Pneumonia is an infection of the lungs that can be caused by the bacteria called pneumococcus. This bacteria can cause other types of infections too, such as ear infections, sinus infections, and meningitis (infection of the covering around the brain and spinal

cord), bacteremia and sepsis (blood stream infection). Sinus and ear infections are usually mild and are much more common than the more severe forms of pneumococcal disease. However, in some cases pneumococcal disease can be fatal or result in long-term problems, like brain damage, hearing loss and limb loss. Pneumococcal disease spreads when people cough or sneeze. Many people have the bacteria in their nose or throat at one time or another without being ill—this is known as being a carrier.

Polio *(Can be prevented by IPV vaccine)*

Polio is caused by a virus that lives in an infected person's throat and intestines. It spreads through contact with the feces (stool) of an infected person and through droplets from a sneeze or cough. Symptoms typically include sudden fever, sore throat, headache, muscle weakness, and pain. In about 1% of cases, polio can cause paralysis. Among those who are paralyzed, up to 5% of children may die because they become unable to breathe.

Rubella *(German Measles) (Can be prevented by MMR vaccine)*

Rubella is caused by a virus that is spread through coughing and sneezing. In children rubella usually causes a mild illness with fever, swollen glands, and a rash that lasts about 3 days. Rubella rarely causes serious illness or complications in children, but can be very serious to a baby in the womb. If a pregnant woman is infected, the result to the baby can be devastating, including miscarriage, serious heart defects, mental retardation and loss of hearing and eye sight.

Tetanus *(Lockjaw) (Can be prevented by Tdap vaccine)*

Tetanus is caused by bacteria found in soil. The bacteria enters the body through a wound, such as a deep cut. When people are infected, the bacteria produce a toxin (poison) in the body that causes serious, painful spasms and stiffness of all muscles in the body. This can lead to "locking" of the jaw so a person cannot open his or her mouth, swallow, or breathe. Complete recovery from tetanus can take months. Three of ten people who get tetanus die from the disease.

Varicella *(Chickenpox) (Can be prevented by Varicella vaccine)*

Chickenpox is caused by the varicella zoster virus. Chickenpox is very contagious and spreads very easily from infected people. The virus can spread from either a cough, sneeze. It can also spread from the blisters on the skin, either by touching them or by breathing in these viral particles. Typical symptoms of chickenpox include an itchy rash with blisters, tiredness, headache and fever. Chickenpox is usually mild, but it can lead to severe skin infections, pneumonia, encephalitis (brain swelling), or even death.

If you have any questions about your child's vaccines, talk to your healthcare provider.

Last updated on 03/26/2014 • CS246005-A

APPENDIX D. RECOMMENDED IMMUNIZATIONS, 2014

E

National Health Observances

Month	Topics	
January	Healthy weight	Blood donation
February	Dental health	Burn awareness
March	Nutrition	Red Cross
April	Autism	Earth day
May	Asthma	Skin cancer
June	Headache	Home safety
July	Eye injury	Firework safety
August	Immunizations	Medic alert
September	Injury prevention	Alcohol and drugs
October	Heart health	Fire prevention
November	Smoking cessation	Diabetes
December	Hand washing	Safe toys

Source: Adapted from National Health Information Center (2011); National Wellness Institute (2011); and Wellness Council of America (2011).

APPENDIX

F

Body Mass Index Graphs

APPENDIX FI

2 to 20 years: Boys
Body mass index-for-age percentiles

NAME _____

RECORD # _____

Date	Age	Weight	Stature	BMI*	Comments

*To Calculate BMI: Weight (kg) ÷ Stature (cm) ÷ Stature (cm) x 10,000
or Weight (lb) ÷ Stature (in) ÷ Stature (in) x 703

AGE (YEARS)

Published May 30, 2000 (modified 10/16/00).
SOURCE: Developed by the National Center for Health Statistics in collaboration with
the National Center for Chronic Disease Prevention and Health Promotion (2000).
http://www.cdc.gov/growthcharts

CDC
SAFER · HEALTHIER · PEOPLE™

APPENDIX F2

2 to 20 years: Girls
Body mass index-for-age percentiles

NAME _____

RECORD # _____

*To Calculate BMI: Weight (kg) ÷ Stature (cm) ÷ Stature (cm) x 10,000
or Weight (lb) ÷ Stature (in) ÷ Stature (in) x 703

AGE (YEARS)

Published May 30, 2000 (modified 10/16/00).
SOURCE: Developed by the National Center for Health Statistics in collaboration with
the National Center for Chronic Disease Prevention and Health Promotion (2000).
http://www.cdc.gov/growthcharts

CDC
SAFER · HEALTHIER · PEOPLE™

Glossary

504 Accommodation Plan An accommodation plan for children who have been identified with learning and other types of disabilities under the Rehabilitation Act of 1973–Section 504

Americans with Disability Act (ADA) The 1990 law that prohibits discrimination against people with disabilities in all areas of public life—jobs, school, transportation, and places open to the public

Bisexual A person who sexually partners with males and females

Body mass index A measure of body fat based on a calculation that involves height and weight

Child Abuse Prevention and Treatment Act (CAPTA) The 1974 law that provides federal funding to states in support of child abuse prevention, assessment, prosecution, and treatment activities

Child protective services agency The name given to a government agency in many states that responds to reports of child abuse

Child Study Team A group of professionals typically employed by a board of education to provide parents and teachers with a variety of learning-related services for the child with special needs

Coordinated school health program A systematic approach to improving the health and well being of all students so they can fully participate and be successful in school

Culture Behaviors and beliefs characteristic of a particular social, ethnic, or age group

Cultural competency The ability to interact effectively with people of different cultures and socioeconomic backgrounds

Cultural diversity The coexistence of different ethnic, gender, racial, and socioeconomic groups within one social unit

Cultural sensitivity Consciousness and understanding of the morals, standards, and principles of a specific culture, society, ethnic group, or race, joined by a motivation to acclimate one's actions with such

Curriculum Content Standards The health knowledge and skills students should know and be able to perform at different educational levels

Emergency care plan (ECP) A plan written for a student who could present a classroom emergency due to a medical condition; it indicates what to do if the emergency happens, the medication to give, and whom to call and should also include a picture of the student

Gay A person who sexually partners only with someone of the same sex

Health literacy Competence in critical thinking and problem solving leading to responsible and productive behaviors

Health People **initiative** The comprehensive, nationwide health-promotion and disease-prevention agenda, revised every 10 years to meet specific health objectives

Heterosexual A person who is sexually attracted to someone of the opposite sex

Homosexual A person who is sexually attracted to someone of the same sex

Individualized Education Plan (IEP) A document mandated by IDEA that defines individual goals for a child with a disability

Individualized Healthcare Plan (IHP) A proposed sequence of actions developed by the school nurse using the nursing process to meet the health needs of a student

Individuals with Disabilities Education Act (IDEA) The 1990 federal special-education law that ensures that all schools serve the educational needs of students with disabilities

Lesbian A female who sexually partners only with females

Licensed practical nurse A nurse who cares for the sick, injured, or disabled under the supervision of a registered nurse or physician; in California and Texas, known as a *licensed vocational nurse*

Morbid obesity The state of being more than 100 pounds above one's ideal body weight; indicated by a BMI over 40

Obese A medical condition in which excess weight negatively affects one's health and life expectancy; indicated by a BMI over 30

Registered professional nurse A nurse who has graduated from a nursing program at a college or university and has passed a national licensing exam

Transgender An umbrella term describing different gender identities that do not match with a person's assigned sex, such as transsexual, transvestite, and cross-dresser

References

Allensworth, D. D., & Kolbe, L. J. (1987). The comprehensive school health program: Exploring an expanded concept. *Journal of School Health, 57*(10), 409–412.

American Academy of Child and Adolescent Psychiatry. (2004). Facts for families: Normal adolescent development. Retrieved March 21, 2011, from www.actforyouth.net/resources/rf/rf_stages_0504.cfm.

American Nurses Association. (1998). *Scope and standards of professional school nu rse practice.* Silver Spring, MD: Author.

Autism Speaks. (2010). What is autism? Retrieved November 10, 2010, from http://www.autismspeaks.org/whatisit/index.php

Bellows, L., & Moore, R. (March, 2013). *Childhood overweight.* Retrieved January 18, 2015, from www.ext.colostate.edu/pubs/foodnut/09317.html.

Berg, F. (2004). *Underage and overweight: America's childhood obesity crisis: What every family needs to know* (pp. 3–33). Long Island City, NY: Hatherleigh Press.

Borkar, R. (2010). Cultural diversity in our schools. Retrieved November 2, 2010, from http://www.buzzle.com/articles/culturaldiversity-in-schools.html

Brain Injury Association of America. (2004). Brain injury in children. Retrieved July 27, 2014 from http://www.bianusa.org/brain-injury-children.htm

Brodeurk, P. (2002). Access to care: School-based health clinics. Retrieved August 30, 2010, from http://www.rwjf.org/files/publications/books/2000/chapter01.html

Bruey, C. T. (2004). *Demystifying autism spectrum disorders: A guide to diagnosis for parents and professionals* (pp. 45–80). Bethesda, MD: Woodbine House.

Centers for Disease Control and Prevention. (2006). Facts about ASD. Retrieved November 13, 2010, from http://www.cdc.gov/ncbddd/autism/facts.html

Centers for Disease Control and Prevention. (2008). Childhood obesity facts. Retrieved November 17, 2010, from http://www.cdc.gov/HealthyYouth/obesity

Centers for Disease Control and Prevention. (2009). Health insurance coverage: Early release of estimates for the national health interview survey, 200d. Retrieved from http://www.cdc.gov/nchs/nchis.htm.

Centers for Disease Control and Prevention. (2013a). National Health Education Standards. Retrieved January 23, 2013, from http://www.cdc.gov/healthyyouth/sher/standards

Centers for Disease Control and Prevention (2013b) *What is child abuse and neglect? Recognizing the signs and symptoms*, retrieved October 31, 2014, from http//www.childwelfare.gov

Centers for Disease Control and Prevention. (2014a) About BMI for children and teens. Retrieved January 19, 2015, from www.cdc.gov/healthyweight/assessing/bmi/childrens_bmi/about_childrens_bmi.html

Centers for Disease Control and Prevention. (2014b) *Elder abuse: Definitions*. Retrieved on February 7, 2015 from www.cdc.gov/violenceprevention/elderabuse/definitions.html

Collins, J., Goodman, R., & Moulton, A. (2008). A CDC review of school laws and policies concerning child and adolescent health. *Journal of School Health, 78*(2), 69–119.

Davidson, T. (2003). *School conflict* (pp. 34–35). New York: Scholastic.

Edmonds, Molly. (2010). *Are teenage brains really different from adult brains?* Retrieved online November 5, 2014, at http://science.howstuffworks.com/life/inside-the-mind/human-brain/teenage-brain1.htm

Garber, B. D. (2010). *Developmental psychology for family law professionals*. New York: Springer Publishing.

Gilbert, G. (2000). *Health education: Creating strategies for school and community health*. Sudbury: MA: Jones and Bartlett.

Grapes, B. J. (Ed.). (2001). *Child abuse: Contemporary issues companion*. San Diego, CA: Greenhaven Press.

Great Schools. (n.d.). School attendance: Issues to consider. Retrieved August 30, 2010, from http://www.greatschools.org/parenting/behavior-discipline/school-attendance-issues.gs/com

Healthy People 2010. (n.d.-a). Retrieved December 9, 2010, from http://www.healthypeople.gov/2020/default.aspx

Healthy People 2010. (n.d.-b). Final review. Retrieved July 28, 2014 from www.cdc.gov/nchs/data/hpdata2010/hp2010_final_review.pdf

Healthy People 2020. (n.d.) Topics and objectives—Objectives A–Z. Retrieved August 10, 2014 from www.healthypeople.gov/2020/topicsobjectives2020/

Klauke, A. (1989). Coping with changing demographics. ERIC Digest Series. EA45. Retrieved November 2, 2010, from http://www.ericdigests.org/pre-9214/coping.htm

Lavoie, R. (2005). *It's so much work to be your friend* (p. 295). New York: Simon & Schuster.

Maslow, A. H. (1943). A theory of human motivation. *Psychology Review, 50*(4), 370–396.

Meeks, L., Heit, P., & Page, R. (2009). *Comprehensive school health education: Totally awesome strategies for teaching health* (6th ed., pp. 4–24). New York: McGraw-Hill.

National Association of School Nurses. (2002). *The use of telehealth technology in the practice of school nursing. Position statement.* Silver Spring, MD: Author.

National Association of School Nurses. (2005). *Environmental impact concerns in the school setting. Position statement.* Silver Spring, MD: Author.

National Association of School Nurses. (2006). Disaster preparedness: School nurse role. Retrieved October 12, 2010, from http://www.nasn.org/Default.aspx?tabid=221

National Association of School Nurses. (2010). Definition of school nursing. Retrieved October 20, 2014, from http://www.nasn.org/RoleCareer/PlanningaCareerinSchoolNursing

National Association of School Nurses. (2011a, revised). *Pediculosis management in the school setting. Position statement.* Silver Spring, MD: Author.

National Association of School Nurses (2011b, revised). *Role of the school nurse. Position statement.* Silver Spring, MD: Author.

National Center for Chronic Disease Prevention and Health Promotion. (2009). Strategies for increasing protective factors among youth. Retrieved August 15, 2010, from http://www.edc.gov/HealthYouth/AdosescentHealth/connectedness.htm

National Center for Chronic Disease Prevention and Health Promotion. (2010). Alcohol and drug use. Retrieved August 13, 2010, from http://www.cdc.gov/HealthYouth/alcoholdrug/index.htm

National Center for Education Statistics. (2009). Indicators of school crime and safety. Digest of Education Statistics. Retrieved September 10, 2010, from http://nces.gov/programs/digest/d09/tables/dt09-052.asp

National Center for Educational Statistics. (2014). *The condition of education, indicator 13, children and youth with disabilities.* Retrieved February 7, 2015, from http://nces.ed.gov/pubs2014/2014083.pdf

National Children's Advocacy Center. (2010). Physical and behavioral indicators of abuse. Retrieved December 17, 2010, from http://www.nationalcac.org

National Health Information Center. (2011). *National health observances.* Washington, DC: Office of Disease Prevention and Health Promotion, U.S. Department of Health and Human Services. Retrieved June 22, 2011, from http://healthfinder.gov

National Institute on Drug Abuse. (2010). *Preventing drug abuse among children and adults: Risk factors and protective factors.* Publication no. 10-7583. Retrieved August 15, 2010, from http://www.nida.nih.gov/prevention.risk.html

National Wellness Institute. (2011). Health observances. Retrieved June 22, 2011, from National Wellness.org

New Jersey Department of Education. (2009). *School health services guidelines* (pp. 1–141). Trenton, NJ: Author. Retrieved from http://www.state.nj.us/education/students/safety/health/services

Praeger, S., & Zimmerman, B. (2009). State regulations for school nurse practice. *Journal of School Nursing, 25*(6), 466–475.

Rimm, S. (2004). *Rescuing the emotional lives of overweight children* (pp. 6–25, 45–51). New York: St. Martin's Press.

Saisan, J., Smith, M., & Segal, J. (2009). Child abuse and neglect: Recognizing and preventing child abuse. Retrieved October 24, 2010, from http://helpguide.org/mental/child_abuse_physical_emotional_sexual_neglect.htm

Saugus.net. (1998). Computer terms glossary. Retrieved December 1, 2010, from http://www.saugus.net/ComputerTerms/

Schwab, N., & Gelfman, M. (Eds.). (2001). *Legal issues in school health services: A resource for school administrators, school attorneys and school nurses* (pp. 499–500). North Branch, MN: Sunrise River Press.

Scudder, L. E. (2006). Pediatric growth and development. In S. M. Nettina (Ed.), *Lippincott's manual of nursing practice* (8th ed.). Philadelphia: Lippincott Williams & Wilkins.

Selekman, J. (Ed.). (2006). *School nursing: A comprehensive text* (pp. 3–21, 28, 45–55, 60, 80, 205–232, 301–320, 391–406, 945–954, 833–860, 1135–1136). Philadelphia: F.A. Davis.

Summerfield, L. (1992) Comprehensive school health education. ERIC Digest. Ten topic areas to be included in any comprehensive school health program. Retrieved from http://www.ericdigests.org/1992-1/health.htm

Trickett, P. K., & Schellenbach, C. J. (1998). *Violence against children in the family and community.* Washington, DC: American Psychological Association.

U.S. Department of Health and Human Services. (n.d.). The Affordable Care Act. Retrieved July 30, 2014, from http://www.hhs.gov/healthcare/rights/

U.S. Department of Health and Human Services, Centers for Disease Control and Prevention. (n.d.). 2014 recommended immunizations for children from birth through 6 years old and 7 through 18 years old. Retrieved June 24, 2014, from http://www.cdc.gov/vaccines/parents/downloads/parent-ver-sch-0-6yrs.pdf and http://www.cdc.gov/vaccines/who/teens/downloads/parents-version-schedule-7-18yrs/pdf

Wellness Council of America. (2011). Health observances. Retrieved January 2, 2011, from http://www.welcoa.org/observances

Wold, S. J. (1981). *School nursing: A framework for practice* (pp. 3–17, 20–29, 39–47). North Branch, MN: Sunrise River Press.

Wolfe, D., & Mash, E. (Eds.). (2006). *Behavioral and emotional disorders in adolescents: Nature, assessment and treatment* (pp. 2–34, 535–540). New York: Guilford Publications.

World Health Organization. (n.d.). Disabilities. Retrieved July 17, 2014 from http://who.int/topics/disabilities/en/

Further Reading

Advameg. (2010). Mainstreaming. Retrieved September 14, 2010, from http://www.faqs.org/health/topics/2/Mainstreaming.html

American Academy of Pediatrics. (2008). Disaster planning for schools. *Pediatrics, 122*(4), 895–901.

American Nurses Association & National Council of State Boards of Nursing. (2013). Principles for delegation by registered nurses to unlicensed assistive personnel. Retrieved July 31, 2014, from www.nadona.org/pdfs/Principles for Delegation.pdf

Bosch, C. (1997). *Schools under siege: Issues in focus* (pp. 5–17, 77–91). Springfield, NJ: Enslow.

Bowman, R. (1994). Cultural diversity and academic achievement. Retrieved November 1, 2010, from http://www.ncrel.org/sdrs/areas/issues/educators/leadrshp/le0bow.htm

Centers for Disease Control and Prevention. (2010). Morbidity and mortality weekly report (June 4, 2010). Retrieved January 18, 2015, from http://www.cdc.gov/mmwr/pdf/ss/ss5905.pdf

Centers for Disease Control and Prevention. (n.d.-a). Body mass index age–percentile charts for boys and girls. Retrieved online, August 27, 2014, from http://www.cdc.gov/healthyweight/assessing/bmi/childrens_bmi/about_childrens_bmi.html

Centers for Disease Control and Prevention. (n.d.-b). Classification of biological agents of concern. Retrieved March 21, 2011, from http://cdc.gov/agent/agentlist-category.asp

Centers for Disease Control and Prevention. (n.d.-c). Head lice information for schools. Retrieved August 4, 2014 from http://cdc.gov/parcites/lice/head/schools.html

Eaton, D. K., Kann, L., Kinchen, S., Shanklin, S., Ross, J., Hawkins, J., . . . Wechsler, H. (2010, June 4). Youth risk behavior surveillance—United States, 2009. *Morbidity and Mortality Weekly Report (MMWR)*. Retrieved November 4, 2014, from http://cdc.gov/mmwr/preview/mmwrhtml/ss5905a1.htm

Faracone, S. (2003). *Straight talk about your child's mental health: What to do when something seems wrong.* New York: Guilford Press.

First Signs. (2010). Autism spectrum disorders. Retrieved November 10, 2010, from http://www.firstsigns.org/delaysdisorders/asd.htm

Kutscher, M. L. (2005). *Kids in the syndrome mix.* Philadelphia, PA: Jessica Kingsley.

Lynch, E. W., & Hanson, M. J. (1992). *Developing cross-cultural competence* (pp. 35–59). Baltimore, MD: Paul H. Brookes.

Mainstreaming. (2009). Retrieved September 14, 2010, from http://www.faqs.org/health/topics/2/Mainstreaming.html

Marin, P., & Brown, B. (2008). *The school environment and adolescent well-being: Beyond academics. Child trends research brief* (pp. 26). San Francisco: National Adolescent and Young Adult Health Information Center.

McLeod, S. A. (2007). Maslow's hierarchy of needs. Retrieved July 29, 2014, from http://www.simplepsychology.org/maslow.html

National Association of School Nurses. (2004). *School health records. Issue brief.* Silver Spring, MD: Author.

National Association of School Nurses. (2014). *Our history. Position statement.* Silver Spring, MD: Author.

National Board for Certification of School Nurses. (2014). *Certification examination for school nurses handbook.* New York: Author. Retrieved August 25, 2014, www.nbcsn.org

Newton, J., Adams, R., & Marcontel, M. (1997). *The new school health handbook: A ready reference for school nurses and educators* (3rd ed., pp. 15–16, 353–364, 371–375). Paramus, NJ: Prentice Hall.

Offit, P. A. (2008). *Autism's false prophets.* New York: Columbia Press.

Pigott, D. C., & Kazzi, Z. N. (2007). Biological agents of concern. In T. G. Veneema (Ed.), *Disaster nursing and emergency preparedness for chemical, biological, and radiological terrorism and other hazards* (p. 404). New York: Springer Publishing.

Russo, C. (Ed.). (2006). *Key legal issues for schools.* Lanham, MA: Rowman and Littlefield Education.

Sacks, A. (2001). *Special education: A reference handbook* (pp. 43–58). Santa Barbara, CA: ABC-CLIO.

Sarasota County Health Program. (2010). Student cumulative health record. Retrieved November 25, 2010, from http://www.sarasota .k12.fl.us/schoolhealth/studenthealthrecordsanddocumentation

Schantz, S. (2010). What's new in the world of childhood obesity? *NASN School Nurse, 25*(6), 288–292.

Schoessler, S. (2002, May 18). Bits and bytes: Technology for the school health office. Paper presented at Bergen County School Nurses Association, Woodridge, NJ.

Selekman, J. (Ed.). (2013). *School nursing: A comprehensive text* (2nd ed., p. 31), Philadelphia: F.A. Davis.

Simons, J. A, Irwin, D. B., & Drinnien, B. A. (1987). Maslow's hierarchy of needs. In, *Psychology: The search for understanding.* New York: West Publishing.

Summerfield, L. M. (1995, October). National standards for school health education. Why have health instruction in the schools? ERIC Digest Series. ED387483. Retrieved September 7, 2010, from http://www.ericdigests.org/1992/health.html

Transcultural Nursing. (2008). Cultural competence. Retrieved November 1, 2010, from http://www.culturediversity.org/ cultcomp.htm

U.S. Department of Health and Human Services. (1997). A research based guide for parents, educators and community leaders (2nd ed.). Retrieved October 10, 2010, from http://www .healthypeople.gov

U.S. Department of Health and Human Services. (n.d.). 2009 national youth risk behavior surveillance report. Retrieved from http://www.cdc.gov/mmwr/pdf/ss/ss5905.pdf

U.S. Secret Service and U.S. Department of Education. (2002). *Threat assessment in school: A guide to managing threatening situations and to creating safe school climates.* Washington DC: Author.

Veenema, T. G., Benitez, J., & Benware, S. (2007). Chemical agents of concern. In T. G. Veneema (Ed.), *Disaster nursing and emergency preparedness for chemical, biological, and radiological terrorism and other hazards* (p. 484). New York: Springer Publishing.

Volokh, A., & Snell, L. (1998). Strategies to keep schools safe. Retrieved October 19, 2010, from http://reason.org/news/ show/1007114/html

Washington State Office of Superintendent of Public Instruction. (2000). Levels of nursing care for student diseases and conditions: Severity coding. Staff model for the delivery of school health services (pp. 8–24). Author.

Zaiger, D. (2000). *School nursing practice: An orientation manual* (2nd ed.). Castle Rock, CO: National Association of School Nurses.

Index